MICHAEL YESSIS

SECRETS OF

RUSSIAN

SPORTS FITNESS

AND TRAINING

FORMERLY SECRETS OF SOVIET SPORTS FITNESS AND TRAINING

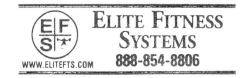

ELITE FITNESS
SYSTEMS
WWW.ELITEFTS.COM   888-854-8806

Secrets of

Russian

Sports Fitness and Training

By
Michael Yessis, Ph.D.

Revised 2008

Formerly *Secrets of Soviet Sports Fitness and Training*, Arbor House, NY 1987

Published by:

Ultimate Athlete Concepts

Michigan USA

2008

For information and to order copies: www.ultimateathleteconcepts.com

CONTENTS

Preface

This book is an update of *The Secrets of Soviet Sports Fitness and Training,* published in 1987. Most of the original information is still applicable today even though a few short sections and comments are somewhat outdated. The bulk of the material is still as good today as it was 21 years ago. With some of the added material, this book becomes one of the best sources of how the Russians developed such great athletes and an effective guide as to what it takes to develop high level athletes.

Rather than rewriting the entire book, sections are added at the end of each chapter as an addendum to update the information. Thus, be sure to read the addendum to get the latest information on changes that have taken place over the last 21 years. In this way you will be getting the latest, most advanced information on the Russian system of training athletes.

Much of the information in the addendums has come from additional conversations with Russian coaches and continued readings of their scientific and coaching journals. The new information can help give you a much better understanding of the entire Russian system of training athletes, which even today is proving to be very successful.

It is even possible to find many American coaches now using Russian methods with great success. This has been confirmed to me through the many positive comments from coaches who have used different aspects of Russian training methods with great success. By reading the updated information together with the original material, you too will be able to experience greater success in your athletic endeavors regardless if you are a coach or athlete.

Note that the use of the term Russian can be used synonymously with Soviet as in the original text. "Soviet" applies to the Union of Soviet Socialist Republics while "Russian" is for the country of Russia, the dominant country after the breakup of the USSR. Thus the terms Soviet and Russian can be used as synonyms. Today, many of the republics that were a part of the Soviet Union are independent and compete under their own flags. Russia is smaller than the USSR but is still very large. Many of the independent republics now excel in certain sports in the Olympic and world championships.

Chapter 1:

How You Can Benefit from Soviet Sports Techniques

If you're like millions of other Americans, vivid images of the 1984 Summer Olympic Games in Los Angeles have been permanently etched in your memory. Whether the sport was track and field, gymnastics or swimming, U.S. athletes never performed with such intensity, such inspiration, and such success. By the time the closing ceremonies brought the games to a close, the American competitors had captured 174 medals. It was a proud moment for this country.

Yet while 140 nations were represented at the XXIII Olympiad, I'm sure you recall that one country was conspicuously absent. The Soviet Union had chosen to boycott the games, and pressured most of its Eastern-bloc allies to stay home as well. As a result, a lingering question nagged at sports fans both during and after the Olympics—namely, were the U.S. athletes on the victory stand so frequently because their Soviet counterparts had remained in Moscow? Or were the American athletes really that good?

These questions may have been debated for years, were it not for an event that took place in the weeks immediately after the Los Angeles games. The Soviet-bloc nations staged their own "alternative" competition—the Friendship '84 Games—in Moscow and several Eastern European countries. And many of the Olympic champions must have felt quite unsettled when they compared the results of the Los Angeles and Moscow meets.

In track and field, for instance, the Soviets outperformed the Western athletes in twenty-eight of forty-one events. In every distance event the Friendship winner was faster than the Olympic gold medalist. Even in the shorter races, the achievements of Los Angeles standouts like Evelyn Ashford (100 meters) and Valeric Brisco-Hooks (400 meters) were overshadowed by the performances of the Soviet stars.

But the painful news was not confined only to track and field. Swimmers from the West did not fare much better. Five world records were broken in the Friendship Games, and forty swimmers there eclipsed the times which won gold or silver in Los Angeles. In the women's 100-meter freestyle, two East German swimmers surpassed the winning time of Americans Nancy Hogshead and Carrie Steinseifer, who had finished in a dead heat for the Olympic gold medal.

Other international meets have put a further damper on our achievements in the 1984 Olympics. In the world gymnastics championships in Montreal in late 1985, U.S. athletes went head to head with their counterparts from the Soviet Union and East Germany. When the medals were tallied, competitors from the U.S.S.R. had won eleven gold, three silver, and two bronze, while the East Germans took home a total of ten medals. And the Americans—who had won the men's gold, the women's silver, and many individual medals in the Los Angeles Olympics—were shut out, capturing not even a single award.

Unfortunately, the bad news for the West has continued. In 1986, in Ted Turner's inaugural seventeen-day Goodwill Games in Moscow, Soviet athletes won 118 gold medals and 241 medals overall, compared with 42 gold and 142 overall for the Americans. As the Associated Press reported, "The games, billed as a battle of the superpowers, was a mismatch, as the powerful Soviets overwhelmed the Americans."

The message was no better when the top swimmers from both East and West competed in the world aquatics championships in Madrid in 1986. The Americans were consistently blown out of the water by their Eastern-bloc peers. The final scorecard showed the U.S. with just five of twenty-six individual events and two of six relays. It was the worst that an American team had ever fared in a major competition, leading the head swimming coach of the U.S. to tell reporters that the swimming program in the States would undergo a complete re-evaluation.

Results like these in international meets have become uncomfortably commonplace for the United States. In almost all sports, athletes from the Soviet Union and other socialist-bloc nations have consistently outperformed Western competitors. The credit for the U.S.S.R.'s unparalleled success lies with the most sophisticated, scientifically based system of training athletes in the world, one that is many years—and in some respects, decades—ahead of the U.S. approach.

As you will learn in this book, the Soviets do many things differently in sports than we do in the West. The East Germans have come as close as any nation to adopting the rigorous Soviet training program, and by fully utilizing this research (as well as some of their own), their athletes have fared exceptionally well in one international meet after another. But even so, no one takes athletics more

3

seriously, no one analyzes sports performances in such detail, no one prepares for international meets more conscientiously than the Soviets. They are constantly developing novel training regimens, innovative equipment, and new competitive tactics.

As you move through this book, the Soviet system may strike you as quite complex. Your mind may boggle when you encounter an array of multisyllabic training approaches—ergogenics, metrology, plyometrics, biomechanics, specialized preparatory exercises, autosuggestion, periodization, cycling, restoration—that have had their origins in the U.S.S.R. Don't let them daunt you. The intent and the outcome of the Soviet approach remain simple: To help everyone in the country, from school-age children to world-class competitors, achieve his or her athletic potential. And they've succeeded remarkably well.

Although the Soviet Union is accumulating the largest body of scientific research on the training of athletes, much of it has been ignored in the West. True, we know and admire the achievements of some Soviet athletes, such as Olga Korbut, Valery Borzov, and Tamara Press. Even so, most American coaches routinely react with skepticism to any training information that filters from the U.S.S.R. to the United States. They seem convinced that it is only propaganda designed to sabotage our own approaches to sports training.

That isn't all. There are also constant claims that Soviet athletes are professionals, supported by the belief here that they are well-paid to train and perform on a full-time basis. And of course illegal drug use is frequently credited (or blamed) for the outstanding performances by Eastern-bloc athletes at international meets.

I am convinced that we're making a terrible misjudgment with this kind of thinking. In fact, it is the many years of Soviet sports research—legitimate research with legitimate aims— that have paid off most handsomely for the U.S.S.R. Soviet training principles and practices have been tested and proven over the last two to three decades. And if these same techniques were put into practice in the West rather than being ignored, I believe that we could immediately raise our levels of performance by helping each of our athletes take advantage of all of his or her talent.

However, there is reason for hope. Fortunately, we can now draw upon the best that the Soviet system has produced. For the past twenty-five years, I have studied Soviet sports theory, research and training as intensively as anyone in the West, and have always been intrigued by how willing their coaches have been to share information that they have developed—if we are willing to listen.

In 1968, I first learned just how accessible the Soviet coaches and their ideas were. I was attending a U.S.-U.S.S.R. track meet in Texas, where I was coordinating a series of week-long seminars with coaches from both countries. During these sessions, I was immediately impressed by how openly the Soviets answered questions asked by the Americans about their training techniques. They were not at all secretive about what they and their researchers had developed. This openness was very refreshing, particularly since most of us from the West were expecting something quite different.

Since then, I have traveled to the Soviet Union four times, most recently in 1986. Whether I was accompanying the U.S. volleyball team or another group of American athletes and coaches, the Soviets were always eager to talk. During one visit, for instance, I stayed in the homes of U.S.S.R. coaches in Moscow and Minsk. They showed me the formal training manuals of their national teams, which I read eagerly. Eventually I realized that once the Soviets get a sense that you're not going to exploit or ridicule them, they are enthusiastically cooperative.

5

Some Soviet coaches have even told me that they want the quality of American athletics to attain levels on a par with that of the U.S.S.R. Their reason is that they wish to continue holding international meets with our teams in the U.S. As one coach said, "If you don't have teams strong enough to present us with a challenge, we're not going to be able to come over to compete against you. And we love coming here . . . we love your culture—and your department stores and clothing shops."

My own knowledge of sports behind the Iron Curtain has come from more than just personal contact with coaches and athletes. I have also spent many years studying scientific sports journals published in the Soviet Union, and learning about the theoretical and applied research that they conduct in many different sports. These journals, incidentally, are not intended for export, but are written for coaches in the U.S.S.R. to keep them up to date on the latest sports research on the country's elite athletes. Thus, they are not doctored for propaganda purposes. Instead, they are ongoing sources of accurate information on the latest in sports practice behind the Iron Curtain, in areas ranging from cardio-respiratory endurance to "speed-strength" training to sports medicine.

As I am proficient in the Russian language, I have translated many of these articles for publication in *Soviet Sports Review,* the quarterly English-language journal I edit and publish for coaches in the West. But except for this American periodical, information on sports research in the U.S.S.R. is not reported on this side of the Iron Curtain, even though athletes here—from the elite competitor to the weekend jogger— could benefit enormously from it.

The Soviets tell me that they devour every bit of information they can get that emanates from U.S. sports researchers. They implement the findings they think are significant, often long before most of our own coaches do.

On occasion, this research by U.S. coaches is carefully scrutinized in Soviet books and journals. A book published behind the Iron Curtain in 1985 objectively evaluated some of the studies done in the West on strength training for high-level swimmers and concluded that their claims were "exaggerated" and "of an especially narrow character." While noting that the dramatic improvements promised by the U.S. coaches may have been "possible in poorly trained swimmers at a low skill level, they in no way apply to well-prepared, high-level athletes." Although the American researchers were promoting the benefits of isokinetic strength training, the Soviets presented data showing an "indisputable advantage" in utilizing free weights and specialized training devices.

Turnabout would be fair play, but you'll rarely — if ever — see American books or journals evaluating Soviet sports research in this way. In fact, most attempts to expose Americans to information gathered by Soviet researchers are greeted with a notable lack of enthusiasm here.

Let me relate an incident that occurred several years ago. I had observed some apparent shortcomings in the running style of one of America's top woman hurdlers. So I wrote to the U.S. Olympic Committee, and included an article from the *Soviet Sports Review* which provided a state-of-the-art analysis of hurdling techniques. I suggested that the article be passed on to the American hurdler, feeling that it could provide her with some pointers to help her improve her style.

Not long thereafter I met this hurdler at a track meet, and asked if she had found the article useful. She looked at me with a surprised expression on her face. "I never received it," she said. In our conversation that day, however, she was intrigued by what I told her about the Soviet research, and she asked to see the study. Unfortunately, someone at the U.S. Olympic Committee had apparently felt that this Soviet study was not worthy of her attention.

What happens when this kind of information does filter down to athletes in the U.S.? The results are often astounding. I have already witnessed a growing number of success stories of Americans whose performances have been dramatically improved once various Soviet techniques have been adopted. In my own consultations with National Football League players, Olympic-level divers, and coaches of the U.S. volleyball squad, I have clearly seen that the approaches developed in the U.S.S.R. can be just as effective with athletes in the U.S.

Consider the dramatic improvement that these techniques made possible in Phil Murphy, who was a lineman with the Los Angeles Rams when I worked with him. Phil was a talented player, but he wanted to be more explosive off the line, and asked for my help. I placed him on some specialized exercises developed in the Soviet Union, including some that were designed primarily to improve his leg strength and acceleration.

The results were exciting. Within months Phil had lost seven inches off his waist. Although he weighed in at over 300 pounds, he had 255 pounds of lean muscle mass—more muscle than any other lineman on the team.

When the preseason began, Phil was a different player than he had been the year before. Because of his hard work with the innovative Soviet techniques, he was able to burst off the line with such speed and intensity that opposing teams consistently had to double-team him to keep him from sacking the quarterback. Ironically, his coaches had difficulty believing that a man weighing more than 300 pounds could develop such swiftness, and thus they were hesitant to play him. But when they did, quarterbacks of opposing teams became instant believers as Phil would nimbly and aggressively bear down on them, play after play. It was wonderful to watch.

The story of Phil Murphy is just one of many dozens that I could tell you. Whether athletes are professional or non-professional, these Soviet approaches have proven effective for Americans.

I recently counseled a woman in her forties who began as a weekend runner but was soon taking her sport seriously enough to enter marathons, including the New York Marathon. However, she ultimately developed leg and back pains that doctors were unable to relieve, which forced her to stop running.

I began working with her in the weight room, and became surprised at how weak her legs were. She had so little muscular strength that while performing a leg-extension exercise, she was unable to lift even 10 pounds. So I decided to place her on a Soviet program designed to build power in her legs. I felt that, in turn, this would relieve much of the strain that was being placed on her back.

I also changed her running style in line with techniques that have been adopted in recent years in the U.S.S.R. She had been a heel-hitter—landing on her heel with the full force of her body weight, jarring her entire body (including her back) in the process. But I recommended that she switch to a "ball-whole foot" approach — striking the ground with the ball of the foot first, and only then allowing the rest of the foot to land on the ground. As a result, the impact of landing was more evenly distributed throughout her body — and the pain in her back and legs subsided. For the first time in her life, she said, she was able to train pain-free.

I am convinced that so many more Western athletes — including elite ones — could benefit from what the Russians have learned. For example, I am often amazed when watching Zola Budd, an outstanding runner who could be even better if her technique were improved. Next time you see her run, notice the flailing of her arms. I believe she could cut a few precious seconds off her times

9

by keeping them close to her sides and synchronizing them better with the rest of her body. Some shoulder and arm exercises developed by Soviet researchers could have an enormous payoff for her.

But what about you? No matter the role sports play in your own life, you can now benefit from many of the Soviet breakthroughs and innovations. Don't let the differences in lifestyle or political systems between the West and the East interfere with your acceptance of what Soviet sports scientists have learned. Whether you hope to participate in the next Olympic Games or merely to cut a few seconds off your time in the five-kilometer races in your community, there is information in this book that you can utilize to reach your personal goals.

So no matter where you currently find yourself, there is something in these chapters for you. Even if your athletic endeavors are limited to swimming a dozen laps each morning, or bicycling a few miles on the weekends, you can get more from your exercise by adopting a sophisticated conditioning program, making use of some psychological monitoring, and learning how to prevent and recover from injuries.

If you take your sports more seriously than this, and are already competing on a college or even a professional level, you will surely notice the glaring differences between the Soviet and the Western approaches to training. In the U.S., for instance, our world-class swimmers have recently moved into the weight room as part of their training program. Our coaches are convinced that big muscles achieved through weightlifting will result in greater speed in the pool — and more medals. But while Soviet swimmers once relied heavily on this kind of strength training, that is no longer the case. Instead, they have replaced it with something new — "speed-strength" techniques.

Under this new system, Eastern-bloc swimmers utilize heavy weights only for six to twelve weeks and then switch to lighter loads and faster movements. The result: More explosiveness in the arms and legs, resulting in even greater speed in the water. Speed, the Soviets have learned, is achieved in (and out of) the weight room through low resistance and rapid execution. No wonder they fare as well or better than we do in international competition in the pool.

Restoration is another area in which Soviet researchers are strides ahead of us. After a rigorous workout, your body may still be feeling fatigued the next day when you head to the track or the training room. But in the U.S.S.R. athletes are now implementing approaches to recuperation that are virtually unknown in the West. Although some of them require special equipment — like Kravchenko pressure chambers and hydro-therapeutic baths — others, such as unique therapeutic sports massage techniques and nutritional supplements, can be utilized no matter what resources are available to you. In the process you will find yourself recuperating more quickly after each training session, in turn allowing you to train harder and thus improve your performance. At the same time, restoration techniques will reduce the number of injuries you experience.

But unfortunately, we in the U.S. continue to be exposed to the Soviet approach to sports only infrequently. I believe that American television does us a disservice in the way it covers major international sporting events, from the Olympics to the Goodwill Games. We rarely see the Eastern-bloc teams (or any other foreign teams) perform unless they happen to be competing against our own national team. The networks are uninterested in featuring anyone but the U.S. athletes.

I hope you will approach this book with more of an open mind. Although there are major political differences between the East and the West, there is much that we can learn from the Soviets in areas like athletics. Fortunately, the secretiveness that permeates so much of Soviet society has not infiltrated the sports world, and this information is now available to us, almost for the asking. Opinions about the Soviet political system should not influence how you view their training methods. This is objective, scientific research, and has nothing to do with politics, "Star Wars," nuclear weapons, Afghanistan, or religious persecution. Instead, it deals with the development of athletic talent — theirs and yours. If you give the techniques described in this book a chance, you may be surprised at how much they will help your own performance and enjoyment, no matter in what athletic endeavor you are involved.

Chapter 1 Addendum

The examples from some of the Olympic Games and world championships described in this chapter are now history. However, the basic premise behind the Soviet (now Russian) system remains basically the same regardless of the fact that the original sports complex has been broken up.

The monies that were originally given to the sports programs are no longer available but yet coaches and athletes continue to be successful. This shows the resiliency of the basic programs that were instituted throughout the nation. It also indicates that the sports (physical education) system developed for the schools continues to remain basically intact in many areas. Understand that the Russians emphasize the teaching of skills and a progression of teaching skills in the elementary and secondary grades throughout the country. This is what enables many youngsters to develop their athletic talent and excel as they become older.

Note that we have nothing like this in our elementary and secondary schools! But, this is one aspect of the Russian program that can help improve our sports greatly. In this case the schools would be responsible for the teaching of skills, which as we know, are not taught or taught as well as they should be in the youth leagues and high school teams. In addition, if this practice was copied from the Russians, the teaching of sports skills would be fairly standardized throughout the nation. Regardless of where the youngster is raised, he would be receiving basically the same education.

In addition, in the United States the teaching of sports skills (technique) to future physical education teachers is practically non-existent. For some reason it is believed that skills are learned while playing games. The Russians believe the opposite. You should master the skills first and then play the game. In my practice I have found that learning the skills first leads to more effective playing and even more enjoyment from the playing.

After meeting and talking to Russian coaches working in the US and in Canada, I have been impressed with their opinions of American athletes. They are truly amazed at the amount of talent that we have and find it hard to understand why we don't develop more high level Olympic and world champions. They are the first to point out that we do not have a system for training athletes and that each coach does his "own thing" with no cohesion between coaches throughout the country.

Many former Soviet coaches who left the country can now be found working throughout the world. There are Russian coaches presently in China, Spain, Argentina, the Arab Republics, Italy, U.S., Canada and other countries. In fact, it can be said that the increased success in many of these countries is due in part to the presence of these coaches. According to them, if we had different aspects of the former Soviet system in place, we would see a world of difference in the development of athletes.

In the last 5-10 years, there are have been some fairly significant changes in the United States in regard to the use of Russian training methods. For example, periodization is now quite common and used in almost all sports based in part on the information in the original text. Periodization is now being applied and experimented with. There is also much more information available on periodization from the Russians especially from the works of Dr. Anatoly Bondarchuk. He is probably the most successful Olympics coach in history. A former Olympic bronze medal winner in the hammer throw, who has a Ph.D. in Sports Science, he trained hammer throwers who won the gold, silver and bronze medals in four consecutive Olympics. No other coach in history has come even close to duplicating such a dominant feat.

I recently translated one of his books, *Transfer of Training* in which there is much dealing with not only periodization but the application of different exercises and how they relate to success in a particular sport. For more information on this book, please visit www.dryessis.com.

Other examples of incorporating Russian training methods include more effective use of general preparatory exercises, plyometrics, and to a limited extent, specialized exercises. There is now better differentiation between general physical preparation (GPP) and specialized physical preparation (SPP) although the latter is, for the most part, still misapplied. We still lag behind greatly in the areas of biomechanical analyses of sports technique, ergogenetics, auto suggestion, cycling of training and especially in restorative measures. More will be discussed on these in the upcoming chapters.

Although the Russians accumulated the largest body of scientific research on the training of athletes in the world, much of it is still being ignored in the West. Many "experts" refute the research done by the former Soviets with statements such as "their statistics do not hold up" or "the research is flawed" etc. What they fail to recognize or look at more closely is the success achieved by the athletes by the research that was done.

As a former professor of physical education (now Kinesiology) I had many discussions with my peers throughout the country about this. Most agreed that the information would be of interest but they were not inclined to research or even read the material or to teach it in the classroom. If it wasn't in the textbook that they used it was considered unimportant. To a good extent this was understandable since the teaching of sports skills and sports training to future education teachers is not a priority in the universities. Simple perusal of college curriculums will show that academic treatment of these topics is practically nonexistent. But yet, in the Russian institutes for future coaches and physical education teachers this was a top priority.

If the universities were serious about training future sports coaches and teachers the professors would have copies of this book, a full set of the *Fitness and Sports Review* journals, *Transfer of Training* by Anatoly Bondarchuk, *Block Periodization* by Vladimir Issurin and *Special Strength Training* by Yuri Verkhoshansky. These journals and books would be considered basic and essential to not only understanding the Russian system of training but also getting the latest information on sports training. Sadly however, it does not appear that most professors will have even seen any of this material in the next few years.

Even the criticism of the statistics used by the Russians is often erroneous. The statistical methods used by them were the most modern in the world at that time. Thus, if we refute what was done then, we should refute all the research done in the United States and the rest of the world prior to the introduction of, as for example, double blind studies. However, we know that this would be a drastic error. The statistical methods may not have been as powerful, but they still provided great evidence and indications of what took place and the probabilities were very high that the results that they found were indeed accurate. More on the topic of research is discussed in chapter 3.

A few words are also necessary here in regard to the belief that the former Soviet athletes succeeded mainly because of drug use and because they were professional athletes. Today, as we learn more about drug use in the United States, it has become obvious that even though the Soviets used drugs, U.S. athletes were also using drugs. And, if we look at the amount of money paid to professional athletes today it becomes clear that we still do not see the world's best performances.

Thus, once again money may be important to stimulate the athlete to train harder to achieve more success, but the money by itself does not make a great athlete. It is the training system that makes the athlete. It is not drugs, money or other enticements. Regardless of your environment or what you are taking in, you must still train. This is the only way one can excel in sport. Thus, as I brought out then and I will emphasize now, the real secret to Russian success is in their training system.

I have been trying for many years to get this message about Russian training methods out to the media, coaches and athletes. Sadly however, the media refuses to look at the training of an athlete or player development. The media appears to be more concerned with sensationalizing drug use or other aspects of a players' life rather than what he or she must do to be great. There are many classic examples of professional sports not using any science in the development or training of their athletes.

For example, in baseball, pitchers and hitters are not scientifically analyzed through the use of high speed taping with frame by frame analysis of their technique. Nor are the coaches learned or trained to be able to recognize what are true errors, what needs adjustment, what corrections should be made and how they should be made based on the tapes. Instead, teams rely on people who "eye-ball" a players' performance and tell them what they can do to become better. This is a very unscientific method and is successful only if it is a lucky guess; most often it is not. But when the athlete achieves even a modicum of success this method is highlighted in the media.

To illustrate, there was a recent article about one of the San Diego Padres pitchers who had a great beginning season but started having difficulty and didn't win a game for over a month. He finally won a game and it was attributed to the minor adjustments made by the pitching coach. His adjustments included having him throw more downward in his release. But yet, science tells us that when a pitcher releases the ball, it is released at an upward angle and gravity pulls it down so that it crosses the plate in the strike zone. If the pitcher released the ball downward, it would hit the dirt before reaching home plate.

But yet, this correction was extolled as a major breakthrough in helping the pitcher achieve success since he once again won a game. Not addressed was if his problem was throwing the ball too high out of the strike zone. Then this correction would be valid. But there was no indication of this since he did not walk many batters during his slump. This is an example of baseball still being in the dark ages when it comes to the application of science in analyzing and improving player performance.

Part of the reason for this may lie in the fact that baseball coaches believe they are already doing everything that can be done to improve player performance. However as I recently found out, their meaning of improving player performance is quite different from the basic understanding. Player development usually means improving the athlete's skills which are specific to his or her sport, that is,

18

their technique. In addition, it means improving or increasing the athlete's physical qualities such as strength, explosive power, flexibility and agility, especially as they relate to the athlete's technique.

By improving skill and the physical qualities specifically related to the skill, the athlete will be able to better carry out his game functions. This means for example, that he will be capable of running faster, cutting quicker and sharper, jumping higher, hitting more powerfully and accurately, etc., depending upon the needs of his sport.

A different definition of player development is understood in baseball. They believe that , "Development is the maturation of the skill that you're bringing into the system. It's the vocal and the physical force constantly around these players during their growth years."

Baseball personnel explain that the team would help hitters be "patiently aggressive." Pitchers would be preached to about "pounding the strike zone", throwing " first-pitch strikes" and commanding the 'outer half' of the strike zone. Passionate words about the changeup would also be spoken."

From these comments it is obvious that player development means teaching strategy and tactics, not improving player abilities in relation to technique or physical qualities. This is even borne out in the comment that "...the primary objective will be simple: let them play baseball. The entry-level staff will do more watching than teaching."

It appears that baseball teams believe that with more playing--even though many of the players have already been playing 12 to 15 years, they will become better players. They believe that by just playing and getting talked to, the player will become better in his skills and abilities. But as the Russians and others have proven through science and practical experience, this does not happen.

Players do not become faster, more powerful or throw harder, through playing. This requires training. It is necessary to work on technique and improvement of the physical qualities specific to the technique. This does not mean general physical conditioning to get in shape to play; this is only a prerequisite to specialized training.

The assumption that athletes already have the needed technical and physical skills is erroneous. I as well as the Russians, have found that all players can be improved in their skills and physical abilities. This is true not only in baseball but in other sports. Because of this, as have the Russians, I have come to the conclusion that all athletes, regardless of their level, can be even better than they are. It took me some time to understand this but it finally came through after reading many Russian biomechanical analyses of world-class performers. There was not a single athlete who was found to be perfect in technique or to have fully developed physical qualities specific to his or her technique.

Although interest in the former Soviet training methods has increased in the US, it has still not permeated the main training centers. Interest is seen with selected coaches, especially strength coaches, who are always looking for an edge in terms of making the athletes stronger, faster and more explosive. However, interest in national organizations that train hundreds of future coaches and strength coaches are still lagging behind in this area. Many of these organizations appear to be more concerned with personal trainers rather than strength coaches who will be dealing with athletes of the future. However, it should be noted that many personal trainers now work with athletes, including professional.

Many of the articles that I translated from the Russian and that appeared in the Soviet Sports Review, later known as the Fitness and Sports Review International, are still as good today as they were the day they were published. The reason for this is that the information has still not been incorporated or acted upon. But yet, this information is very useful and can prove to be valuable in improving the performance of many athletes. Thus, I strongly recommend that if you are interested in more sound, scientifically based information, you should read some of the research and training articles in various sports in the back issues.

Another area that has not seen change in the US is in technique analysis. But yet, this is one of the most important areas that can greatly improve an athlete's performance. Understand that there are two major ways of improving an athlete's performance. One is through better technique, the other is through improved physical qualities, especially those that relate specifically to his or her technique. Improved technique is one of the tenets of the former Soviet system of training athletes, especially in the area of specialized training.

For example, the main criterion for a specialized exercise is that it must duplicate the technique seen in execution of the sports skill. In other words, you must develop strength in the way that it is displayed in the sport. This includes not only the same motor pathway but strength must be developed in the same range of motion and the muscle contraction regime must be the same. You develop strength together with proper technique which not only improves technique, but also performance, because of the combined elements (often known as the conjugate system of training).

To help coaches in this area I have written several books dealing with technique analysis and how technique can be improved in different sports. Coaches who have used these books have seen tremendous improvement in their athletes. To

21

my knowledge they're the only books that deal extensively with what constitutes good technique and how it can be improved. These books include *Explosive Running*, *Explosive Basketball Training*, *Explosive Golf*, *Women's Soccer: Using Science to Improve Speed*, *Explosive Tennis* and *Build a Better Athlete*. The latter book contains analyses of the basic skills of running, jumping, throwing, hitting and kicking.

As I bring out in the original Secrets book, using the techniques and information presented can improve your performance and enjoyment no matter which sport you're involved in. The information presented has proven of value many times over. I can guarantee that you will see positive results from incorporation of some or all of the methods that are presented in this book.

Chapter 2:

The Role of Sports in the Soviet Union

Within the walls of the Kremlin, sports are perceived as more than just fun and games. For decades, athletics and fitness have been an integral part of the Soviet political system itself.

A little history is in order here. Shortly after the Russian Revolution of 1917, Communist party leaders recognized physical exercise as a means of improving the strength of the country and its people. By promoting exercise, they believed that the nation's productivity could be enhanced through a decline in fatigue on the job and absenteeism due to illness. Fitness was also recognized as a way to keep the population healthy and prepared for military combat. As one Soviet sports authority has written, "The ultimate goal of physical culture [sports] in our state is to prepare the younger generation for a long and happy life, for highly productive labor for the benefit of society, and for defense of their socialist homeland."

The usual birth date of Soviet athletics is given as 1918, for in that year a cross-country run was held in Moscow, thereby becoming the first postrevolutionary sports event. By 1921, more than 150 sports clubs had been formed in the U.S.S.R., and some 6,000 physical education instructors had been trained. In 1928, the First Workers' Spartakiad was held in Moscow, commemorating the tenth anniversary of Soviet sports programs, with thousands of athletes participating in events in twenty-one sports.

In the pre-World War II period, emphasis was placed on expanding the number of sports facilities in the U.S.S.R. Between 1931 and 1940, their ranks grew fourfold, and major stadiums were built in Moscow, Leningrad, and other cities. Many of these older facilities are still in use, with crude equipment and dilapidated gymnasiums commonplace in many parts of the nation. Nevertheless, despite their age, they are still quite capable of producing excellent athletes.

During World War II, the U.S.S.R. credited the physical fitness of its soldiers—and the general public—with helping its people withstand agonizing months of hunger and fatigue. Marshal Konev, a Soviet commander, wrote, "Only physically fit people can stand the strain of heavy fighting, can march long distances under perpetual bombardment, and quite often have to start fighting at the end of a long march. We owe it primarily to the sports organizations that Soviet people were training and had imparted to them such qualities as courage, persistence, willpower, endurance, and patriotism."

Soviet sports programs were vigorously revitalized in the postwar era, and they have grown steadily thereafter. Particularly since 1952, when the U.S.S.R. first began participating in the Olympic Games, the result has often been Soviet dominance in world athletics. The nation's success in international competition has been a means of generating national pride and uniting people from all parts of that vast country. At the same time, leaders in the Kremlin see victories at the

Olympics as propaganda tools for boosting the image and prestige of the Soviet system: In essence, a win for athletes from the U.S.S.R. is perceived as a victory for socialism, especially when those triumphs come at the expense of capitalist countries.

Physical-fitness programs now affect the life of almost every Soviet citizen. True, there is nothing in the U.S.S.R. comparable to Little League or Pop Warner football, which involve so many thousands of American children in sports. But fitness behind the Iron Curtain continues to be considered an integral component of a well-rounded individual, and a way of keeping the population as a whole physically and psychologically healthy. Thus, beginning on the playgrounds of pre-schools, children have the opportunity to develop their strength, speed, and stamina as part of organized school and recreational programs. In physical fitness tests that are part of a program called GTO ("Readiness for Work and Defense of the U.S.S.R."), children enthusiastically compete for pins and buttons earned by running, jumping, and throwing. The primary aim of GTO is to get the entire population of the country active in some kind of sports activity.

Exercise periods two to three times per week are as much a part of Soviet schools as mathematics and science, with organized recesses and "physical culture" breaks a carefully planned part of the curriculum. For those youngsters who demonstrate considerable sports skills, and who have particular physical and psychological qualities, an elaborate system has been created to develop their talents. Because the Soviets do not have the broad base of athletic participation that a Little League might provide, the GTO program makes special efforts to seek out potential stars and steer them toward developing their raw talent to the fullest. Across the U.S.S.R., there is a "talent search" for those children possessing all-around physical abilities. Their present and future body size and qualities are evaluated, and the parents are often looked at as well in order to determine a child's genetic inheritance and what he or she may become.

Despite myths to the contrary, the Soviets do not "rob the cradle" to create their athletes, selecting children almost at birth to mold into the sports stars of the future. However, a sophisticated approach is utilized to develop the talents of children wherever these exist, usually starting no earlier than age nine (except for swimmers and gymnasts, who may begin a little earlier).

When a youngster is singled out as a candidate for athletic achievement, he or she is offered the opportunity to attend a sports school for children, beginning at an age deemed appropriate for that sport (see Table 1). These special schools play a critical role in the nurturing and development of Soviet athletes. And although it's not mandatory that the selected children go to this school, parents and youngsters usually agree to do so, for obvious reasons. In the U.S.S.R., the high-level athlete fares better in life and enjoys fringe benefits not available to the average worker. Not surprisingly, parents often encourage their children to become athletes.

These sports schools—and there are thousands of them in all parts of the country—include the same academic subjects as regular elementary and secondary schools in the U.S.S.R. Their only distinguishing feature is the outstanding coaching they provide the children. The Soviets firmly believe that by ages eleven and twelve, youngsters are best able to acquire athletic skills. If skills aren't learned during these years, it may be too late for children ever to develop the proper foundation. For this reason, some of the nation's best coaches are assigned to children at this formative age level.

TABLE 1: Age for admission to children's sports schools

Sport	Age (yrs)	Sport	Age (yrs)
Acrobatics	8-9	Biathlon	10-11
Boxing	12-14	Skiing, ski jumping	10-11
Freestyle wrestling, classical wrestling	10-12	Track and field	11-12
Volleyball, basketball	10-12	Swimming	7-9
Water polo	11-12	Table tennis, tennis	7-9
Cycling	12-13	Badminton	10-12
Gymnastics, rhythmic	7-8	Sailing	9-11
Gymnastics, sports		Diving	8-10
Boys	8-9	Handball	10-12
Girls	7-8	Archery	11-13
Rowing, canoes and kayaks	11-13	Soccer	10-11
Rowing, academic (skulls)	10-11	Figure skating (ice skating)	7-9
		Fencing	10-12
Equestrianism	11-12	Weightlifting	11-12
Ice skating	10-11	Chess, checkers	9-12
Skiing cross-country	9-11		
Skiing, slalom, giant slalom, downhill	8-10	Hockey, ice and field	10-11

In a child's initial months and years in a sports school, the emphasis is on all-around training—running, jumping, throwing, kicking, and some weightlifting—rather than on a particular sport. During this period, youngsters become comfortable with their bodies and how to use them, and learn basic coordination which they can build upon in the years ahead. They also develop some of the psychological qualities necessary for training. And while there may be some organized games in which they participate, there is no emphasis on competition at this stage; in fact, coaches who push the children to win, rather than to build skill, are chastised and may even lose their jobs.

About a year after entering the sports school, each youngster's progress is evaluated, and a decision is made as to whether he or she will continue, or return to a regular school. Those children who stay may eventually begin competing for one of the sports clubs that have been formed in all the Soviet republics, regions, and cities.

These schools and clubs produce the athletes who will eventually be promoted up to the next level—namely, the "specialized" children's sports schools, where Olympic reserves are trained, or to the Schools of Higher Sports Mastery, attended by the nation's top athletes, who compete in international meets. Unlike in the U.S., where we really don't know who will be our Olympic stars four, eight, or twelve years from now, the Soviet Olympic teams of the future are already training together in schools designed largely for that purpose.

At these higher levels, there are separate schools for each sport. The youngsters are trained on a multiyear plan, moving into more complex training as they get older. Athletes develop more rapidly in some sports than in others, and as Tables 2, 3, and 4 show, there are variations in the ages at which they are likely to peak.

But the national GTO complex is there even for the youngsters whose athletic talents do not approach Olympic status, and the program continues all the way up to age sixty. It is divided into six age categories, and each concentrates on a different level of skill development.

The youngest children (ages seven to nine), for example, are part of the "beginning" level, where the focus is on mastering specific motor skills through executing simple bodybuilding and coordination exercises (see Figures 1 and 2 for examples of typical exercises). During each ensuing plateau— ages ten to thirteen ("Level 1"), fourteen to fifteen ("Level 2"), and so on—the aim is to further improve athletic preparation and skills. In adulthood, GTO attempts to maintain the health of the population through routines and exercise, using not only barbells but also simple apparatus as illustrated in Figures 3 through 6.

TABLE 2 Age ranges of sports success (men)

	First great success	Optimal Capabilities	Maintaining high results
Event	*(yrs)*	*(yrs)*	*(yrs)*
Track and field			
100 m run	19-21	22-24	25-26
800 m run	21-22	23-25	26-28
10,000 m run	22-24	25-27	28-29
High jump	19-21	22-24	25-26
Javelin	21-23	24-27	28-29
Swimming	14-17	18-22	23-25
Sports gymnastics	18-21	22-25	26-28
Wrestling	19-21	22-26	27-32
Weightlifting	19-21	22-26	27-32
Boxing	18-20	21-25	26-28
Academic rowing	17-20	21-25	26-28
Basketball	19-21	22-26	27-30
Soccer	20-21	22-26	27-30
Figure skating (ice skating)	13-16	17-25	26-30
Cross-country running	20-22	23-28	29-32
Ice skating	18-19	20-24	25-28
Hockey	20-23	24-28	29-32

TABLE 3 Age ranges of sports success (women) of sports

Event	First great success (yrs)	Optimal capabilities (yrs)	Maintaining high results (yrs)
Track and field			
100 m run	17-19	20-22	23-25
800 m run	19-21	22-25	26-27
High jump	17-18	19-22	23-24
Javelin	20-22	23-24	25-26
Swimming	12-16	17-20	21-23
Sports gymnastics	15-17	18-22	23-26
Basketball	16-18	19-24	25-27
Figure skating (ice skating)	13-15	16-24	25-28
Cross-country running	18-20	21-25	26-28
Ice skating	17-18	19-24	25-28

At each plateau, participants in the program have certain norms toward which they're expected to strive. If they reach those goals — that is, run the 100-meter dash or the 1,000-meter cross-country event in a particular time — then they are awarded pins (see Tables 5, 6, and 7). Each of these events is intended to build qualities like strength, flexibility, speed, and endurance. Along the way, the GTO program instills an appreciation for fitness and an understanding that these physical skills may someday be needed for the defense of the country.

TABLE 4

Mean age of finalists in the XXIII Summer Olympic and XII Winter Olympic Games

Event	Age (yrs)
100-400 m run (men)	23.4
100-400 m run (women)	23.4
Jumps (men)	23.7
Jumps (women)	23.4
Throws (men)	26.7
Throws (women)	26.2
Track and field	26.3
Sports gymnastics (men)	24.8
Sports gymnastics (women)	18.6
Diving (men)	22.2
Diving (women)	20.2
800-1,500 m run (men)	24.3
800-1,500 m run (women)	24.4
5,000-10,000 m run (men)	27.3
Sports walking, 20 km	29.3
Cross-country races (men)	27.4
Cross-country races (women)	27.1
Ice skating (men)	25.1
Ice skating (women)	23.5
Academic rowing (men)	25.2
Academic rowing (women)	24.1
Swimming (men)	20.1
Swimming (women)	17.5
Classical wrestling	25.7
Freestyle wrestling	25.7
Boxing	22.4
Basketball (men)	24.6
Basketball (women)	23.6
Soccer	24.8
Decathlon	25.1
Pentathlon	25.2

TABLE 5 Beginning-level "Preparatory Start"

Exercise	Units of measurement	For silver pin	For gold pin
Shuttle run, 3x10 m	sec	10.0	9.5
30 m run from a high start	sec	6.0	5.5
Throwing a tennis ball for accuracy	number of hits	1.0	2.0
Cross-country without consideration of time	m	300.0	500.0
Multiple hops	m	10.5	12.5
Rope climb	m	1.5	2.5
Walking on skis	km	1.0	2.0
Swimming	m	12.0	25.0
Obstacle course	points	7.0	9.0

*On this and the following pages, the norms for the early levels of the GTO program are listed.

Though the GTO complex involves nearly all age categories, Soviet athletes have other opportunities for developing physical fitness outside the program. They can take advantage of the growing number of exercise rooms and swimming pools that are now being built at factories and office sites. These exercise facilities are used almost around the clock, from seven in the morning to well past ten at night. Exercise breaks have replaced coffee breaks, and organized teams have been formed for people at all levels, from assembly-line workers to the highest ranks of the military and the KGB.

The Soviets remain convinced that exercise breaks several times a day can improve productivity in the factory while enhancing physical and mental health. If you are a seamstress, for instance, an exercise program would be designed specifically for you that is intended to reduce fatigue in the body parts you use on the job, and to give some movement to those that remain completely inactive while you are working. Similar types of programs are designed for other occupations— welders, secretaries, assembly-line workers, and so on. By promoting exercise and sports among the average citizen this way, the Kremlin also believes it is effectively occupying people's time and is thus successfully combating some of the country's social ills, particularly alcoholism.

TABLE 6 Required exercises and norms for the first level of the GTO complex for boys 10-11 years of age

# in order	Exercise	Units of measurement	For silver pin	For gold pin
1	30m run	sec	5.8	5.2
2	Long jump with an approach run	cm	310	340
3	High jump with an approach run	cm	95	105
4	Throwing a tennis ball	m	30	35
5	Swimming without consideration	m	25	—
	Swimming 50 m	min, sec	—	1:20
6	Ski chases for 1 km:	min, sec	8:00	7:30
	Regions of no snow, riding a	min	16	15
	or cross-country without	m	500	1000
7	Pull-ups on the high bar	number of times	3	5

People in the U.S.S.R. exercise in other ways as well. As in the United States, there's now a jogging craze. Track-and-field journals there have regular sections devoted to jogging— or as the Soviets call it, "running for health" Books by Kenneth Cooper, one of America's running gurus, have been translated into Russian, and have been widely read by joggers. And for those behind the Iron Curtain who like aerobic dancing, copies of the *Jane Fonda Workout* are circulating, and women wear Western-style leotards and leg warmers while exercising.

TABLE 7 Required exercises and norms for the first level of the GTO complex for girls 10-11 years of age

Number in order	Exercise	Units of measurement	For silver pin	For gold pin
1	30m run	sec	6.0	5.4
2	Long jump with an approach run	cm	260	300
3	High jump with an approach run	cm	85	95
4	Throwing a tennis ball	m	20	23
5	Swimming without consideration of time	m	25	—
	Swimming 50 m	min, sec	—	1:30
6	Ski chases for 1 km:	min, sec	8:30	8:00
	in regions of no snow, riding a bicycle 5	min	19	18
	or cross-country without consideration of	m	300	500
7	Rope climb with use of the legs	m	2.5	2.8

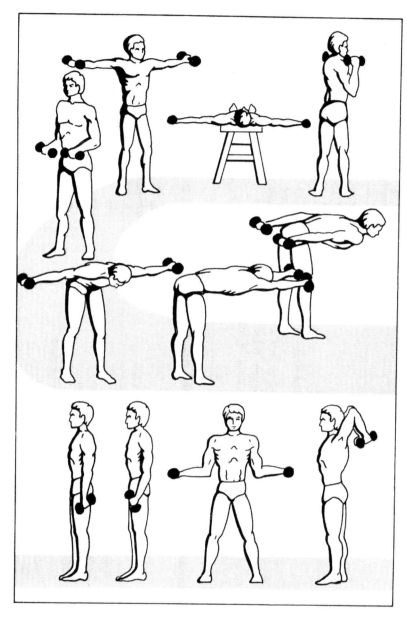

Figure 1. At the beginning level of the GTO
program, boys perform exercises like these.

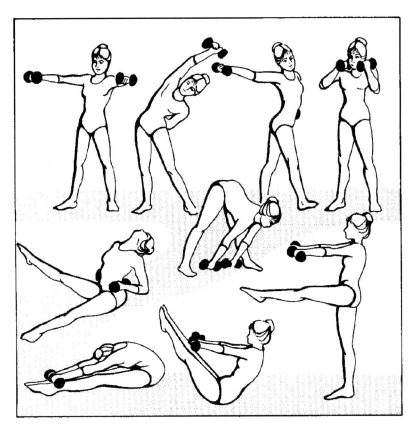

Figure 2. At the beginning level of the GTO program, girls perform exercises like these.

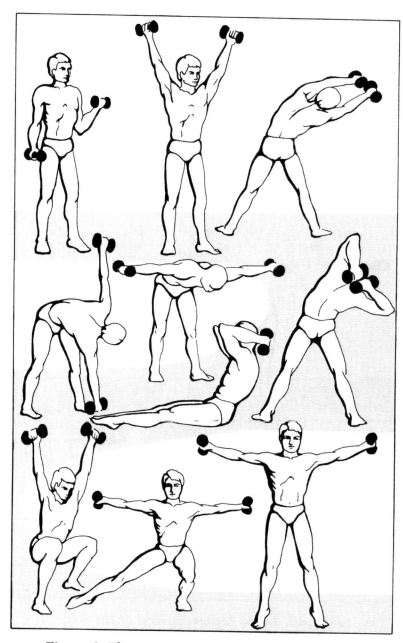

Figure 3. These exercises, and those in Figures 4,
5, and 6, are examples of the types of routines
performed by adults in the GTO program.

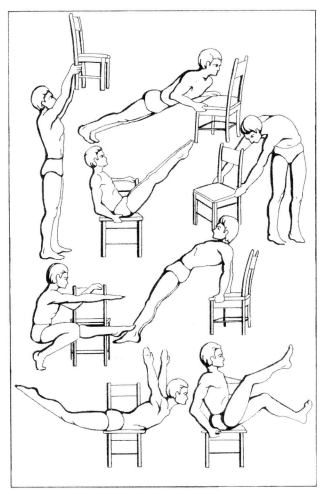

Figure 4. Everyday props like a chair (and a pole in Figure 5) are used by adults to maintain their fitness in the GTO program.

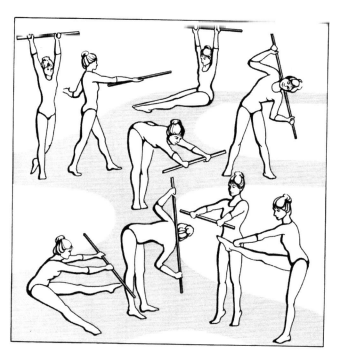

Figure 5.

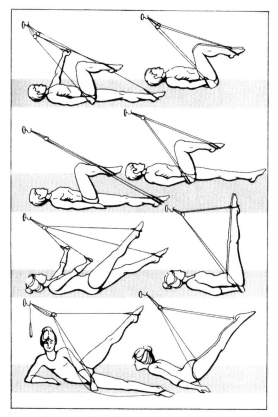

*Figure 6. These all-around body-conditioning
exercises are performed in the U.S.S.R. with a
piece of equipment similar to one popular in the
U.S.—Joe Weider's Body Shaper.*

39

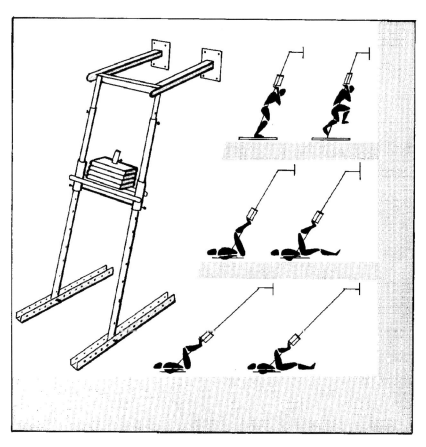

Figure 7. This unusual piece of Soviet equipment can be used in various ways for different effects. Exercises can be done in a standing or a lying position, and the angles can be changed to work the body in different ways.

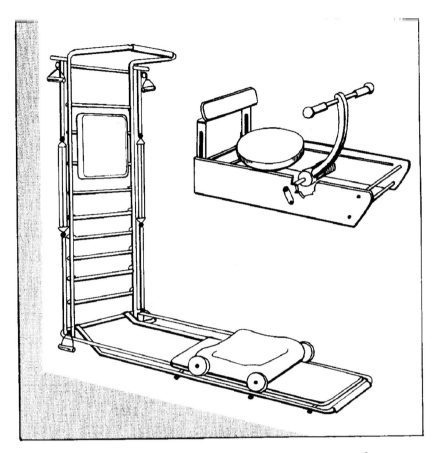

Figure 8. This Soviet exercise apparatus can be adapted in a variety of ways to work the total body. Figures 10 and 11 show some of the applications of this device.

Though Soviet exercise rooms for the average citizen can't compare to our own glitzy, mirror-covered health clubs, they are beginning to be equipped with some multistation exercise machines and stationary bicycles. The most popular equipment in Soviet gyms includes barbells, dumbbells, and kettlebells, as well as the more complex devices illustrated in Figures 7-10. Though kettlebells fell out of popularity in the U.S. several decades ago, the Soviets find them to be enormously versatile, allowing the individual to grab them by the handle, and twist, spin, throw, and catch them. The kettlebell provides a greater range of motion than the barbell (see Figures 11 and 12).

To develop fitness programs for both the public and serious athletes, hundreds of scientists in the U.S.S.R. are involved in full-time research into all aspects of physical well-being. At the National Scientific Research Institute of Sports Culture in Moscow, for instance, the "department of maximology" conducts studies primarily on the nation's elite athletes, with the help of an array of sophisticated equipment in its laboratories, and develops new methods of strength and power training and techniques for psychological preparation for competition.

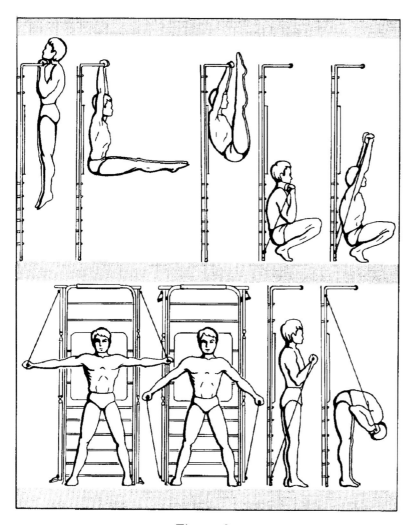

Figure 9.

The research the athletes participate in becomes part of their training program. And these top-flight athletes are the first to put the findings of these studies to the test. Their training schedules and performances are analyzed by a team approach that involves many scientists—from physiologists to biomechanics experts to psychologists to physicians. The Soviets believe that all of an athlete*s actions and qualities are interrelated. Thus, all the different components that contribute to his or her performance are analyzed simultaneously. When this approach is used, the improvements seen in Soviet athletes are often extraordinary. The United States has nothing to compare with it.

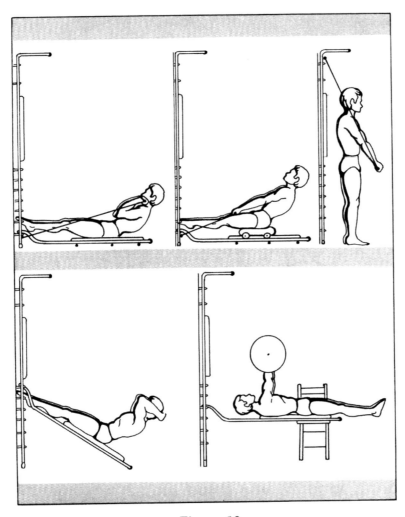

Figure 10.

Interestingly, many of the best Soviet sports researchers were once top-flight athletes themselves. They have been recruited from the athletic ranks not only for their research skills but also because of the belief that they have definite advantages over the "pure" scientist, who lacks the concrete experience to understand the athlete and his problems.

In addition to the National Scientific Research Institute of Sports Culture in Moscow, every republic in the Soviet Union has its own physical culture institute. At these facilities, serious (but not necessarily elite) athletes are examined, analyzed, and evaluated in ways similar to (but often not as intensively as) the studies under way at the National Scientific Research Institute. These athletes are knocking on the doors of the national teams, and the help they receive at the institutes is often enough to elevate them to championship status.

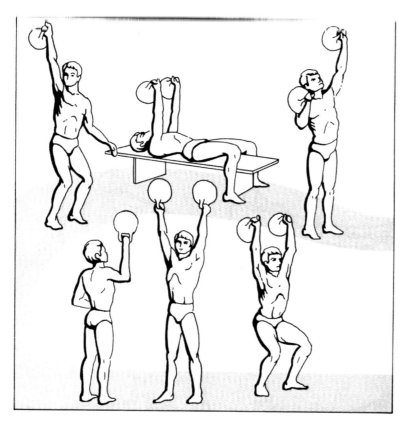

Figure 11. Kettlebell exercises are popular in the U.S.S.R., including those illustrated above for the muscles of the shoulder girdle and knee-joint extensors.

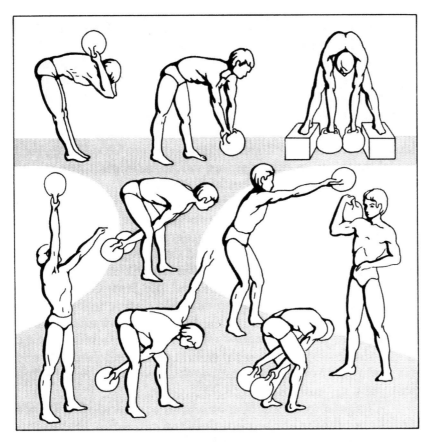

Figure 12. These kettlebell exercises work on the muscles of the spine and the posterior surface of the thighs.

There are facilities at each physical culture institute for nearly every sport. Hockey has its own department, with training rinks, workout rooms, and research labs. The swimming department has its own pools and other training facilities. There are similar departments and resources for volleyball, handball, soccer, track and field, and so on. Wood shops and metal shops are on the premises, too, to build whatever equipment is required by coaches and athletes.

But non-athletes, including young children, are not overlooked in the serious research process. In fact, as much time is spent preparing the training programs for school-age children as for world-class athletes, and thus even preschoolers do not escape the scrutiny of the Soviet Union's sports scientists.

Research breakthroughs behind the Iron Curtain have given Soviet children an enormous head start in many areas of competition. For instance, in the U.S., an American Academy of Pediatrics position paper—citing fears of interfering with bone growth—opposes weight training for preadolescents, and discourages maximum lifts until ages sixteen or seventeen. But that's not the case in the U.S.S.R.

A large body of Soviet anatomical/physiological evidence now shows that prepubescent children *can* safely lift weights —and so they do. From ages nine to thirteen, Soviet children demonstrating potential in weight training begin a general conditioning program with light weights that eventually leads them into specialized routines. The research has examined everything from growth-related epiphyseal disks to heart-circulatory function, and has shown that, rather than causing injuries, the Soviet approach produces better athletes.

Practical applications of sports research like this eventually touch the lives of nearly every citizen of the U.S.S.R. And although facilities like tennis courts and basketball hoops are not yet commonplace in every neighborhood in the Soviet Union, that is rapidly changing. As of today, there are many more sports facilities and opportunities for competition available for American children and adolescents, from grade school through college, than in the U.S.S.R.; but as community swimming pools, for example, become more widespread behind the Iron Curtain, entire families are encouraged to take up water sports, promoting family cohesiveness as well as good health. In the workplace, too, as exercise equipment becomes increasingly available, it is accessible to workers willing to pay a nominal fee (that is, a dollar a year) to join the factory sports club.

And what about the Soviet coaches? Are they as finely tuned and trained as the athletes with whom they work? In the post-World War II years, there was a scarcity of well-trained coaches in the U.S.S.R., and men and women with interest but minimal experience in sports often found themselves coaching some of the nation's top athletes.

Today, however, the development of coaches in the Soviet Union is a scientific, well-planned undertaking. Unlike the U.S., where colleges turn out physical education teachers— some of whom become coaches without any additional specialized training—the U.S.S.R. has developed programs designed specifically to transform young men and women into skilled athletic instructors. Space in these programs is limited, and competition for admittance is keen. All applicants must be serious athletes themselves, and they are required to take rigorous four-day entrance exams in subjects ranging from physics and chemistry to biology and mathematics. Those who make the grade then undergo four to five years of a tough, scientifically oriented curriculum in one of the country's physical culture institutes, which culminates with academic examinations that last for days.

Throughout this educational process, these coaches-in-training keep themselves physically fit, spending about half of each day maintaining their athletic skills at competitive levels. They are also often the subjects of research, learning about sports while having their own performances analyzed.

The men and women who move successfully through this rigorous program become high-level coaches; those who don't become teachers. In the Soviet bloc, then, one does not become a coach on a whim; rather, coaching is viewed as a career that requires special training and education. Every five years, in fact, the coaches return to the physical culture institutes for a semester to receive refresher courses.

Once coaches are ready to begin working with athletes, they are assigned to any region of the country where they're needed. Their placement will depend on factors such as their own abilities and the sport in which they specialize. If they end up working with the nation's most elite sports performers, they will be assigned only a few athletes at a time, thus allowing for ample individual attention. The ratio of world-class athletes to coaches would make Americans envious: it is usually no more than seven to one, and in certain sports (for example, track and field, swimming, gymnastics), the ratio is often four or five to one.

Even for athletes who are not world-class, enough coaches are available to permit some individual instruction. A typical track-and-field club will have seven or eight coaches— one for sprints, one for middle distances, one for throwing events, and so on. By comparison, a typical track-and-field coach at a U.S. university has thirty to sixty top-level athletes under his wing, who are competing in twenty to thirty different events; with ratios like that, each athlete is on his or her own most of the time, getting little personal instruction on the subtleties of training, conditioning, performance, and competition.

I recall a conversation I overheard between one of America's top college track coaches and some of his Soviet peers. The Soviet coaches were asking how his teams consistently produced such great runners. But rather than crediting his own training techniques, the U.S. coach simply responded, "We have so many runners that if they're not great in the one hundred or the two hundred meter dashes, we'll put them in the four hundred. We'll find a place for them, I really don't do much coaching of them at all; they're already good. I just psych them up."

The Soviets, disbelieving, continued to seek information about how he trained his athletes. But the U.S. coach simply responded, "I'm not keeping any secrets from you—because I don't have any. I just don't do much with them at all."

This dialogue reflects a belief prevalent among U.S. coaches—that athletes have innate talent, that they are "born" and can't really be "made." With an attitude like this, a lot of talent is wasted in the U.S. The Soviets, however, know that they can't afford to treat their own athletes this way. They don't yet have the enormous pool of talent to draw upon that U.S. coaches do. Consequently, in the U.S.S.R. much more energy is expended on actively training athletes to reach their full capabilities, and, as I have noted, when talent is spotted, it is fostered and nurtured.

As part of the support network for the athletes and coaches, the Soviets have the world's most highly trained and versatile sports physicians, whose expertise extends far beyond the treatment of injuries. Early in their medical careers, after their internships are completed, these young doctors spend time at the physical culture institutes, where they become completely familiar with how athletes train and the skills involved in competing in various sports. Ultimately, these physicians specialize in a particular sport and become thoroughly immersed in what the sport demands from its athletes. Thus, when an injury occurs, they can almost immediately identify its cause because of their exhaustive knowledge of what athletes must go through in that sport.

Not long ago, I spent some time with a Soviet sports physician at an international track meet. He specialized in caring for track-and-field athletes, while also working with athletes from other sports in the off season. At the meet, he and I were watching the high jump, and after an American jumper had made several practice and competitive jumps, the physician said to me, "If he keeps jumping like that, he's going to wind up with an injury. Watch his approach and takeoff carefully."

At first I couldn't see anything wrong with what the American was doing. But as I continued to watch, I could finally see what the Soviet doctor was talking

50

about a subtle error in form. In fact, about six months later, that same high jumper developed a leg injury that forced him out of competition for a while. I was amazed at the way in which this physician was able to look at an athlete perform and accurately predict that an injury would occur.

Given such sophistication, it is not surprising that the Soviets are so far ahead of the competition, no matter what the sport. Even so, American coaches today rarely ask me, "How do the Soviets train? Are their training programs different from ours? Do the coaches have certain skills that make them more proficient than us?"

Instead, drug abuse by Eastern-bloc athletes is typically raised in the West to explain why they so often beat us. Rumors about the Soviets' use of illegal substances have gradually been accepted as "fact" by many of our most prominent amateur sports officials.

Although this issue will be dealt with at length in Chapter Ten, I think it's important to set the record straight here. Yes, some Soviet athletes have used— and still may be using—steroids—but only in small amounts and at carefully chosen times in their training schedule. When used, steroids are taken early in the season to help the athlete gain bulk and strength and, in some cases, for recuperation. But the doses are kept so small that the body's own ability to produce testosterone (the male hormone) is not affected. Because illegal drugs are not used by the Soviets in the months before competition, drug-testing programs at international meets have detected abuse of illicit substances only once or twice among Soviet athletes—far fewer times than among Americans.

It is clear to me that drugs have never been the reason for the Soviets' success. It is the method of training that deserves most of the credit. In fact, as one coach told me, any athlete who abuses drugs by taking large amounts has to train even harder to overcome the negative effects of the illegal substances—including a greater tendency toward injury and a detrimental impact on muscle elasticity.

If you have any doubts about whether drug use is still prevalent in the Soviet Union, look closely at some of their athletes. Their hammer throwers, for instance, do not have the huge muscle development that you would expect from steroid use. In fact, in one sport after another, the Soviet athletes are slimmer and trimmer than they were in the past. Even their weightlifters are a far cry from champions of earlier times like Vasily Alexeyev, who weighed about 350 pounds in his prime; today, Alexeyev's counterparts tip the scales at up to 80 pounds less, without any of the abnormal overdevelopment that drugs can cause.

You may recall the Press sisters—one a discus thrower, the other a shot-putter. In the 1950s they were among the first women who excelled in international competition, and thus they received considerable media attention. There was a widespread feeling in the West that these Soviet women were using drugs that gave them more of a masculine than a feminine appearance. However, I met one of the sisters and her Soviet physician at an international track-and-field meet at Stanford University, and they succeeded in allaying my doubts completely.

I observed that though this talented young woman was huge, she had none of the muscle-mass development and definition nor the excessive body hair that one expects from drug use. She looked soft and fat, not muscular. Having worked with many talented female athletes in the West, I could see nothing obviously different in the Press sister to indicate that she was using drugs. As I built up a personal relationship with the doctor over a number of years, he confided that all the rumors about the Press sisters—(such as, "Were they really men who had undergone operations?")—were untrue. "They're all female," he told me one afternoon, "and they always have been/' He also refuted effectively the speculation about massive drug use by the sisters. And since I had built up such a strong rapport with this physician over time, I had no reason to doubt him, particularly since what he told me was later confirmed independently by a number of Soviet coaches whose objectivity I also trusted.

Over the years, I've learned that many other charges lodged against the Soviet sports system are also untrue. For instance, there have long been claims that the elite athletes in the U.S.S.R. are "professionals"—paid by the government to train year round. According to this theory, these athletes have only one job—namely, to train for and perform in international meets.

Where does the truth lie? It is a fact that the Soviets have developed a sophisticated multiyear program for their elite athletes. For instance, a potential Olympic competitor will be placed on a long-range, detailed program to guide him or her toward international success. Talented volleyball players might find themselves on a nine-to-twelve-year plan, with specific intermediate goals to be met along the way.

But the Soviets do not have "professional" athletes as we know them. It is true that when an athlete is in the military, he may be placed on a team like the Central Army Club, where he is allowed to spend nearly all his time training or competing. His situation is exactly like that of Stan Smith, who was allowed to play tennis while he was in the military.

But aside from the relatively few Soviet athletes who are members of the army, the remainder train with the many sports clubs throughout the U.S.S.R,, and draw no salary for doing so. Like most of their American counterparts, they have jobs that support themselves and their families, although they may be permitted time away from work for training and traveling to meets.

On one of my trips to the U.S.S.R., I was at a stadium in Minsk, waiting to talk to one of the Soviet coaches. As I sat in the grandstand, I noticed a number of high-level athletes entering the stadium and heading for the locker room. Some wore military uniforms, others those of the police. There were some in casual civilian clothes, and others wearing ties and coats. They were some of the U.S.S.R.'s athletes from all walks of life, getting ready for their daily workouts, after which they would return to their jobs. They certainly did not fit the stereotype of a "professional" athlete.

There are also rumors that the Soviet Union pays bonuses to athletes who set world records. Although I have been able to confirm that such bonuses do exist, they are paid rarely, and then only for record-breaking performance.

As already mentioned, I have stayed in the homes of the coaches during my visits there. In many conversations, they have confided to me that most athletes are *not* paid extra for training and competing. In my own research during my trips behind the Iron Curtain, I have learned that some athletes in the major sports — specifically soccer and hockey — have been paid for their outstanding achievements. As I see it, that's not much different from the money available for "amateur" athletes in the U.S. who compete in major sports such as track and field. They are sometimes so highly paid to compete and to endorse products that Carl Lewis, Mary Decker Slaney, and Edwin Moses are among our youngest millionaires.

So the Soviets remain committed to sports research and the international rewards and prestige it can produce. Even so, coaches in the U.S.S.R. told me on a recent trip that they think their nation's preoccupation with the arms race is holding back their sports program from advancing even further and faster. One of them said, "Your President is messing us up, because when he builds up your military machine, it forces us to spend money on ours. And that's taking money away from our sports budgets." (Needless to say, we use the same arguments, insisting that the Soviet arms escalation is channeling money away from other priorities here.) Still, in spite of such complaints, the sports system in the U.S.S.R. remains unparalleled. And it is the sophistication and excellence of this system—not drugs or money—that deserves the credit for the success of the Eastern-bloc athletes. For that reason, I believe the approach to athletics behind the Iron Curtain is worthy of our serious attention, particularly if we wish to be competitive with the Soviets at the international level, as well as in helping our average citizen become and stay fit. And that's what this book is all about.

Chapter 2 Addendum

The material presented in this chapter needs few additions. The original information can still be used to advantage especially for identifying youngsters with potential. Also very valuable is the classification system for athletes according to levels of achievement. Russian coaches have been surprised that the U.S. does not have any system or organizational structure to classify levels of performance and training. There is no system of ranking athletes from the very earliest years as there is in Russia. As a result it is hard, if not impossible, to compare athletes from different parts of the country and even between, Division 1, 2 and 3 schools. In addition, it is hard to know what kind of training they have been exposed to.

It should be emphasized here that the Russians had to develop an athlete identification system. They did not and to this day do not have a broad sports base as exists in the U.S. In fact, there is no country in the world at this time that has as broad a base of athletes as in the U.S. Because of this, the Soviets had to identify those with potential and then develop them into high level athletes. The entire system of training was based on the concept of making an athlete perform better and be able to compete on a world class level.

In comparison, reliance in the U.S. appears to be on numbers. Because of the great number of athletes that participate in sports, especially in the more popular sports, the laws of chance dictate that a high level athlete will evolve, similar to cream rising to the top in natural milk.   They often rise to top not so much because of the coaching, but in spite of the coaching. Success is often based more on what they gained from multiple coaches and what they did on their own in practice. For example, most professional athletes today have personal trainers in addition to those on the team. Also, genetics and early maturation often play major roles in achieving success in the young years.

In speaking with Russian coaches who are familiar with what takes place in the U.S., they are intrigued by the great talent pool that we have. They shake their heads in wonderment thinking about what they could achieve with such a broad talented base. According to the Russian coaches, if we applied a little science to our training and had a more structured system of training athletes, no one in the world would come close to us in competition.

Russian coaches also point out how in the former Soviet Union and to a good extent now, there are sports clubs, schools and training centers in which talented athletes participate. They often train together for weeks, months, and in some cases, years. For example, Bondarchuk recalls summer camps in which the top throwers in the country participated, together with some of the top coaches in the areas of biomechanics, physiology, psychology and other disciplines involved in training. All of the coaches worked in conjunction with one another.

Only now are we seeing rudiments of such trainings in the U.S. as for example with long distance runners. Some of the best long distance runners live and train together in one place. The major difference from what the Russians did is in the coaching staff. Top experts are not in attendance (at least according to the reports received). Their progress and achievements are for the most part, due to the running, especially hard running and pushing one another to go faster and/or further.

A major striking difference in the training of Russian and American athletes is that youngsters in Russian are given a great deal of technique (skill) training. They have many instructors to teach basic skills from the very earliest years. Much of the technique work is done in the elementary and secondary schools and then emphasized and improved upon in the sports schools and in the clubs. The Russians believe that technique is the most important factor to be mastered in the early years. They found that youngsters are best suited for technique (skill) learning from ages 6-12. Skills such as running and jumping are well formed by the age of 11-10. But this does not mean that it cannot be improved in later ages. It just takes longer and becomes increasingly difficult with each passing year.

In regard to strength training, instead of putting the youngsters on exercise programs to develop strength and other physical qualities, youngsters spend considerable time learning how to execute the exercises. For example, in the sport of weightlifting, skill (technique) learning lasts one-two years! In the process of learning they become stronger, but strength is not the key factor being trained, technique is. As they develop and perfect technique, the youngsters are then capable of making greater progress in the handling of heavier and heavier weights when they pass puberty . At this time technique is well learned and the athletes are able to use it to their advantage with the heavier weights and when doing specialized strength exercises.

In the U.S., the opposite happens. Coaches and teachers often take it for granted that youngsters already know how to run, throw, jump, kick, etc. and as a result, spend more time playing and teaching strategy and tactics. They do not emphasize the teaching and learning of technique. Lip service is given to learning technique. If you examine how skills are taught it will be obvious that it is of a very limited and cursory nature and only taught for a week or two out of the season.

For example, in the youth leagues, there is only a few weeks of practice prior to the first game. Thus, some technique work is done at this time, but because of the inability to repeat the repetitions a sufficient number of times to truly master the technique, the youngsters begin competition with poor or inadequate technique. This is seen even in national youth championships! It is easy to spot poor technique in running, throwing, etc. with 11-12 year olders. Their form may be acceptable when they are 6-7 years old, but not during puberty or after.

In the area of strength training, emphasis in the U.S. is usually on how much weight can be lifted—not on how well the exercise is executed. Exercise technique is taught in one to two sessions and then attention is given to how much strength can be displayed. Many weight rooms even have records posted to challenge each athlete in how much he can lift. This results in many injuries that soon do not allow the athlete to do exercises such as the squat, good morning and overhead press. In fact, poor technique is one of the major complaints of many college and professional team strength coaches.

It should also be brought out that most of the sports technique work in the U.S. is done by mothers and fathers who typically base their teachings on their own experiences or from reading a book. But, there are few if any books that have in-depth analysis of the sports skills or even complete descriptions of what takes place in execution of the skill. These well meaning parents may have played the sport, or participated in a weight training program, but this is no guarantee that they understand what occurs in execution of the skill.

As mentioned earlier, in the elementary schools there is little to no skill teaching. There is mostly play with the main objective being to have fun and enjoyment. But what is often not understood is that in order to have "fun", (really satisfaction and enjoyment) you must be able to execute the skill. The better you execute the skill the greater the satisfaction and enjoyment. This is analogous to a job in any workplace. You want (need) your boss to give you precise instructions on doing a project, piece of construction, confronting someone, etc. so that you know the expectations and will be satisfied when the job is done correctly. Without clear instructions on how to do the task, you are unsatisfied because there is no way to perfect the project.

There is still a major discrepancy between the qualifications of Russian and American coaches to teach skills, from the elementary to the professional levels. Most Russian coaches are trained in this area so they are capable of teaching it whereas in the U.S., future physical education teachers and sports coaches are not even taught basic skills in the universities. They may be exposed to them as for example, in one-two class periods on running, throwing and hitting but this is far from being adequate to truly understand what is involved in basic skill execution and how it should be taught. Because of this, it is common to find school staff workers (not teachers) filling in empty coaching positions—not because of their expertise but as a necessity to field a team.

In regard to Russian equipment, it should be noted that the use of kettlebells is now increasing in popularity in the U.S. Although kettlebells are often touted as being needed in the training of athletes, few Russian athletes are seriously involved in kettlebell training. Athletes use kettlebells for many different exercises and there is even a contingent of athletes who participate in kettlebell competition. Thus, the kettlebells play a valuable role and can be used in the training of athletes as well as the average fitness buff. But they do not constitute a major part of the training.

It is necessary to emphasize once again the seriousness and depth to which the Russians go to develop and learn about each sport. As brought out in the original text, each sport has its own department in the physical culture (coaching) institutes. It is here that they carry out much research into training methods, exercises specific to the sport and so on. In the U.S., there is nothing comparable.

We often hear American researchers criticize Soviet research, but yet they cannot even come close to replicating the success achieved from the Russian research in developing new and effective methods of training and evaluating athletes and training programs. The only exception may be in the endurance sports and then only partially. It is easy to criticize old research by comparing it with the latest methods of doing research. But if the research is evaluated on what was state-of-the-art at the time it was done, we would see that much of the research was more than adequate and valid.

Perhaps one of the reasons for misunderstanding Soviet research is that once a finding is substantiated by other studies and proven in practice, details are no longer reported in following studies. It is accepted as a universal "truth" and is usually well known by students, coaches and of course the professors. It's analogous to the law of gravity--It is accepted and not re-proven in each study that makes mention of it. The 'truth' is well accepted.

Perhaps most importantly is that Russian research produced results. In the U.S., research is too often contradictory or incomplete because it is based on a poor understanding of the topic. Also there are too many studies dealing with one

61

small aspect that lends very little if anything to understanding the complexity of the total problem or the study is based on false premises. More will be said about research in the universities in the next chapter.

Before closing, it is necessary to take a quick look at the Russian system of training as it exists today. The Russians have remained a power house in athletics despite the great changes that have taken place. Sports are no longer government subsidized the way they were earlier and many sports schools have been disbanded. Many former republics are now independent nations but are still producing outstanding athletes who may have been competing for Russia.

The Russians, despite many of these changes, still turn out great athletes. This is testimony to the great system of training that they developed, especially now that money is no longer a major factor. Of course money is still very important and without it one would be hard pressed to have any kind of athletic training program in any country. The point here is that even with a massive decrease in the amount of money that was available not only to the research institutes, the physical education institutes and sports schools, the Russians are still capable of turning out great athletes.

Thus, as I have brought out many times, we have not looked at the Russian system of training. This is where their success lies. The media plays up the "fact" that they were professional and used drugs, rather than looking at their training programs. Only today is there some interest, albeit only a little, in the Russian system of training athletes. Those who have used the information available through my translated articles, books and writings about the Russian system and from listening to Russian coaches in the U.S. at clinics, are seeing great success. They want even more information about Russian methods and how they can be used to further improve athletic performance. What is especially surprising is that most of the information that is available, even though it may be 20-30 years old, is still brand new in relation to the training methods used in the U.S. This point has also been brought out in the books by Yuri Verkhoshansky (*Special Strength Training*), Anatoly Bondarchuk (*Transfer of Training*) and Vladimir Issurin (*Block Periodization*). These books have been translated into English and are now available.

As mentioned earlier, a big difference between the U.S. and Russian training systems is in the role of technique. It is difficult for most Americans to accept that technique improvement can enhance competitive performances as much as, if not more than, greater strength or conditioning. As a result, coaches ignore teaching and perfecting technique especially in youth and for specialized strength training.   That they don't spend more time on technique may be explained by the fact that most coaches do not understand technique to the level needed in order to effectively teach it or to develop specialized strength and explosive exercises (conjugate training). Such exercises must duplicate what occurs in skill execution if they are to have positive results.

In the annual training program in Russia, the pre-competitive period is made up of mainly specialized exercises that duplicate what occurs in execution of the skills in competitive play. The exercises imitate or duplicate a portion of the total technique involved, usually a specific key joint action, which when mastered, is then incorporated into the total skill to perfect it.

In the future I hope more books will be written on technique in different sports in addition to mine. As a result, more coaches will be able to learn more about skill technique and incorporate it into their teaching and training. It should be noted here that even the most popular professional teams in the U.S. do not do any specialized training.   Any technique work that is done is done visually without the use of sophisticated video and computer analyses. But analyses by eye are impossible unless the athletes technique is first recorded on tape and then looked at frame by frame.

Even though there are computer analysis programs available, they do not offer true technique analysis. Instead they give a comparison of one performer with another noting the differences between them. They are descriptive not analytical. Understand that when looking at videotape frame by frame, it is still necessary to know the mechanics of the execution. It is necessary to know the why's and wherefores of each joint action, what makes it effective, how the total skill or a portion of it can be improved, and so on.

Instead, professional, collegiate and high school coaches still rely on only their eyes to see what the athlete is doing. This is a physical impossibility because the eyes cannot see the actions that occur in execution of any basic skill. The action is too fast, and there are too many things to look at simultaneously. For example, position and action of the knee, foot, hips, arm, posture, etc. in running. The eyes cannot even see as much as what is recorded with a typical video camera. The eyes see approximately ten images per second, while the video camera captures approximately 30. Once captured, the video camera images can be looked at frame by frame or at slow or regular speeds.

The brain cannot recall the exact movements seen in each of the frames that the eyes recorded. It is physically impossible! Only the more outstanding characteristics of the performance will be retained. Thus, looking at an athlete perform visually is good for gross major errors that may occur in the backswing (preparatory) or follow through actions, but not for the key actions that occur in the power (execution) phase that are most important on the highest levels of performance.

This is obvious in most sports. For example, how can a throwing coach analyze what a pitcher does with his "separate" body movements or what occurs in the hips, shoulder, elbow, etc. without high shutter speed videography? How can a tennis coach analyze all of the actions that occur in a tennis serve or in any of the groundstrokes? How can a swimming coach know the exact movement pattern of the arm under the water? It is impossible. The only thing the coach can see is the beginning and ending, not the heart of the skill. This is why most corrections that they make are made on the initial stance or on the follow through. It is rare if ever, to see any corrections made of what happens in the power phase of the skill.

Similar situations exist in almost all sports. For example, in golf, corrections are made in the stance, grip, backswing and follow through, rarely in the actual downswing. In football, there is no analysis of the quarterbacks throwing actions or of his movement skills if he is a scrambler. Nor is there analysis of the running or defensive backs or receivers in their running and cutting. But yet, a little time devoted to correcting running and cutting technique can prevent hamstring and other injuries and most importantly, improve the athletes speed and quickness. These physical attributes are the key to getting free of an opponent or to be able to keep up with and overtake an opponent.

Similar situations exist in almost all sports. For example, in golf, corrections are made in the stance, grip, backswing and follow through, rarely in the actual downswing. In football, there is no analysis of the quarterbacks throwing nor of the running or defensive backs or receivers in their running and cutting. But yet, a little time devoted to correcting running and cutting technique can prevent hamstring and other injuries and most importantly, improve the athletes speed and quickness. As should be well known, these latter two physical abilities are the key to success in these positions.

Many coaches continue to believe that player performance is due to genetics and cannot be improved except through strategy and tactics. This is a shame. It shows how sports in the U.S. and some other countries are still guided by myths rather than by science and effective training methods.

As the Russian coaches keep telling me—the U.S. has great talent but does not have the training system to develop the talent. Instead we travel to foreign countries looking for more (better?) talent. For example, if you look at most professional baseball teams you will see that many if not most, have up to 50% foreign players!

Once again it is important to reemphasize the role of technique in execution of game skills and when performing strength exercises. This was and remains the main Russian priority from the very earliest years in the development of athletes. All other factors are considered secondary. This belief and practice is so deeply entrenched that it is taken for granted by Russian coaches and scientists. This is why when discussing specialized exercises, skill execution, strength training or other aspects of training, technique is not highlighted—it is assumed that the reader already knows the technique of the sports skill or strength exercise. It is not necessary to reiterate it!

As previously mentioned the teaching and study of technique does not have high priority in the U.S. This includes the teaching of basic and advanced skills and exercises. For example, I have found that with high school players and even many collegiate players, it takes up to 1-2 months to correct what they were taught or that they learned in the earlier years when it comes to execution of strength exercises. Once they begin to execute the exercises correctly, they begin to see great improvement in their performance not only in strength but game performance. In talking with these athletes it is obvious that the coaches used how much weight they can handle as the determining factor for doing the exercise, not technique.

In regard to athletes who have back or knee problems, it has been found that most often they are due to improper technique when executing strength exercises such as the squat and/or deadlift or when running with the heel hit. With proper technique in these and other strength exercises, and/or correct running technique, the athlete experiences tremendous improvement in his performance.

If you desire more information on technique of execution of various strength exercises, read, *Kinesiology of Exercise* or see the DVD, *Exercise Mastery*. These are the only two sources that go into extensive detail on how an exercise should be best executed and why. These sources bring out all the nuances of the exercise and what happens when you make changes in grip, stance, etc. or execute the exercise in a different manner. For technique of sports skills see *Build a Better Athlete*.

Chapter 3:

SOVIET SPORTS RESEARCH: What it has taught the Russians

On one of my visits to the Soviet Union, I was accompanying the U.S. volleyball team to an international tournament. On a particularly chilly early morning, I found myself awake before dawn, unable to go back to sleep,

I decided to get out of bed and jog before the team members themselves had awakened. I put on my running clothes and stepped out into the darkness at about six in the morning, expecting to find myself alone at that hour. But I was wrong. The Soviet volleyball squad was already outside, preparing for a game that was not scheduled to begin for another three hours.

The athletes were not warming up with a volleyball, but were loosening up with some light calisthenics, as well as just talking to one another and listening to their coach. As I jogged by them, there was no doubt in my mind that they would be ready for the game later that morning. I couldn't say the same about the Americans, however, who were still tucked in their beds and wouldn't arise for another hour.

Later that day, I asked the Soviet coach what his team had been doing in the predawn hours. "Our players were relaxing their bodies and their minds," he told me. "It was nice to be out in the cold country air."

A number of other times during that stay in the U.S.S.R., the Soviet's approach to sports amazed me. But the more one learns about the sports system in the Eastern-bloc nations, the less surprising it becomes. As the previous chapter emphasized, the Soviets have developed their own body of sports research, on which their training and competitive techniques are based. And judging by their success in international meets, one must agree that their efforts have been worthwhile.

This chapter describes specific ways in which Soviet researchers approach their studies in the laboratories and on the athletic fields, and report on what they have learned along the way. The human body in competition has never been examined as exhaustively as in the U.S.S.R. This research is pursued with the same intensity—and with the same governmental support—as research seeking cures for cancer and heart disease. And the sophistication of the sports research is made possible by equipment that was unheard of only a short time ago.

For example, when Soviet scientists want to study the running style of a particular athlete, they use high-speed (sometimes three-plane) cinematography to track his or her every motion. They also hook up the athlete to instrumentation that measures all parameters of movement. He or she wears special shoes equipped with force and time receptors, and runs on a pressure-sensitive "electrified" track. Seismo-graphic recording devices, not unlike those used to measure earthquakes, are also activated on the track.

With these devices in place, the researchers are able to determine the rhythm and cadence of the runner's style, the time and duration of contact with the running surface, the amount and direction of force at contact, airborne time, displacement of the body's center of gravity vertically and horizontally, and displacement of the center of gravity of the extremities during the various phases of running. Then, by comparing such measurements with a model of the "perfect runner," coaches can make precise recommendations about how the athlete's style can be changed to improve performance.

At various periods in their training program, elite athletes are tracked in ways that have never been attempted in the U.S. While training on the athletic field, they might have their heart rate monitored with a "cardioleader" that records information on a second-by-second basis. This detailed information about the heart is instantly telemetered to the laboratory, where an exercise physiologist analyzes it, and, if necessary, radios back specific instructions to the athlete.

Other physiological functions, such as ventilation rates, can be monitored in similar ways. In fact, twenty-three different components of blood chemistry can be traced by taking small blood samples before, during, and after workouts.

Just how extensive can this research become? I was amazed by a recent Soviet journal article that analyzed precisely what takes place in the sprinter's body in the fraction of a second after the starter's gun is fired. For instance, in the elite athlete, 0.10 to 0.18 second elapses before the body is actually set in motion, and in that time the sound waves from the gun enter the ear and turn into nerve impulses that eventually lead to a motor reaction. As the runner pushes out of the blocks, the greatest amount of effort—a force up to 100 kilograms (220 pounds)—is executed in the rear leg, whereas the front-block effort measures no more than 70 kilograms (154 pounds). And the data went on and on.

New approaches to research and monitoring are under constant development in the U.S.S.R. In recent years, weight-lifters have had the trajectory of their lifting movements analyzed with a cyclographic device. There are also air tunnels to evaluate the style and form of alpine skiers and ski jumpers. For divers, their height at takeoff can now be monitored in the minutest detail with new equipment and their speed during flight and upon entering the water can be precisely measured.

Many of these analyses are conducted when athletes are performing at their maximum, including during certain competitive meets. The Soviets have learned that the physiological, biomechanical, and psychological changes that occur when performing maximally in competition are different than those one sees during training.

Back in the research labs, film libraries are maintained not only of Soviet athletes, but also of elite performers from other nations, taken during international competition. Before a particular meet, these movies are reviewed, and analyses are made of how rigorous the competition will be and how to carry home the gold. As part of the psychological training for that competition, the Soviet athletes will be made to visualize racing, jumping, throwing, or playing against other world-class performers—and to see themselves consistently finishing ahead of them.

In the U.S., our own video and) film technology has made it possible for many athletes to view themselves in action. But unfortunately, videotapes of over two hundred fields (or frames) per second are necessary for precise analysis, and equipment this sophisticated is very expensive and thus not commonly available. To compound the problem of proper analysis, most athletes don't know what to look for when they do see themselves on videotape or film. They haven't been taught how to pinpoint the strengths and weaknesses in their form as their bodies proceed through their particular athletic event—and there aren't enough experts around to help them.

So even though video and film technology in general is more advanced in the West than behind the Iron Curtain, the Soviets make better use of the expertise they do have. Soviet coaches who work with athletes in throwing events, for instance, are fully trained to help them understand exactly what they see on the screen—from the planting of the forward leg, to the eccentric contraction of the medial rotators of the hip joint, to the maximal stretching of the abdominal wall's rotational muscles, to the wrist-joint flexion and hand pronation that occur as the object is released. Every movement is analyzed in detail.

Research in the U.S.S.R. is published and widely distributed throughout the country to allow the findings of one scientist or coach to be utilized immediately by others. *Theory and Practice of Physical Culture* is the main scientific sports journal published there, respected throughout the world for its quality and credibility. There are also monthly journals for each of the more popular sports like track and field (priced at the equivalent of forty to fifty U.S. cents), and yearbooks for swimming, tennis, weightlifting, soccer, wrestling, and rowing that give all coaches access to the latest research and other pertinent information.

As a result, every researcher and coach knows what his or her peers are doing, and there are comparatively few professional jealousies that get in the way of the wide dissemination of this information. By contrast, I've found that there is much less sharing in the U.S. Coaches here tend to be protective of whatever training approaches they may use, and are generally reluctant to let others know what they're doing.

In the U.S.S.R., many types of researchers take part in the evaluation of an athlete's typical workout, with every exercise studied meticulously to determine its precise benefits, and even when it should be performed for maximum advantage. For instance, scientists have concluded that certain exercises once routinely performed by sprinters really do little but build bigger muscles. Instead, the Soviets have narrowed the training exercises down to a handful that sprinters should be concentrating on, rather than routinely going through a half-dozen others that may not count on the day of the race.

How does this compare to what occurs here? In this country, athletes tend to adhere to the same exercise routines that have been used for many years. Any departures from the schedule occur only when an athlete is attempting to peak in the days just before competition.

Sports scientists behind the Iron Curtain have also found that athletes can benefit from participating in sports other than the one in which they specialize. By doing so, they can tap a broader array of physiological skills, as well as take advantage of a psychologically relaxing diversion. As a result, it's common in Moscow and other Soviet cities for wrestlers, for example, to play twenty minutes of basketball as part of the warmup of their day-to-day training sessions. Likewise, weightlifters often play volleyball as a companion to training in the weight room.

How sharply this differs from American thinking! In the U.S., we believe that the way to be a good runner, for instance, is to run, run, and then run some more. Run longer, run faster, but run. The Soviets, however, now know that during certain periods of the training program, there are other sports that can be used to help make a runner quicker and more flexible, thus developing the all-around physical qualities needed to be a champion.

I recall when the Soviet wrestling team came to the U.S. several years ago for meets with our own elite wrestlers. The American coaches asked their counterparts from the U.S.S.R. to conduct a clinic that athletes from both countries could participate in. The Soviet coaches agreed, and invited the Americans to join them in a typical day's workout.

The teams accompanied one another to a nearby college, where the Soviet coaches asked for some basketballs. Their wrestlers then began playing full-court basketball in the gymnasium, and the Americans joined in. But as they ran from one end of the court to the other, the U.S. wrestlers gradually began dropping out from fatigue. Finally, after about twenty-five minutes, the Soviets moved on to a series of push-ups, sit-ups, and other calisthenics that lasted another fifteen minutes, with the Americans again falling by the wayside. Once these exercises were completed, and as the Americans were trying to catch their breath, the Soviet coach announced, "Okay, now it's time to wrestle!"

For the Americans, the pre-wrestling workout had been exhausting. But in the U.S.S.R., basketball is routinely used as a warmup activity to get the body's juices flowing and to help the wrestlers condition themselves for their own sport. The U.S. competitors had never seen anything like it.

Soviet research has also developed techniques—particularly strengthening exercises for both muscles and joints—for reducing the number of injuries their athletes suffer. Even among weightlifters, who routinely bear the strain of enormous poundage, bodies are so finely tuned that injuries to their joints, ligaments, tendons, and muscles occur much less frequently than in the past.

Another new approach to emerge from the Soviet sports research labs is called "modeling." Using computers to analyze information accumulated over many years, the Soviets help their young athletes work toward a world record that they may be capable of setting in five, ten, or more years, In essence, the computers are able to predict the kinds of physical qualities and performance levels that will be necessary to compete on a world-class level in the future.

In this highly technical analysis, a complete array of performance characteristics is taken into account: psycho-physiological qualities, properties of the nervous system, sensorimotor factors, and so on. Then, with this model in hand, coaches can devise detailed, multiyear training programs aimed at reaching specific performance goals, while also continuously updating them as new information is accumulated.

Imagine how valuable this kind of information is. Of course we already know today's world record in the 100-meter dash, but the Soviets have developed ways to determine what that record is likely to be in 1990, 1995, and thereafter. At the same time, they can project the precise bodily skills and measurements that an athlete will need in order to compete with the best many years from now, and how he or she should train now to reach those goals.

So while it's nice to say, "I want to be a champion" the Soviets have created unique ways to help their athletes become one. Adolescents are not placed on training programs aimed at breaking today's records; instead, they adopt specially designed regimens that can help them approach the records most likely to exist when they reach their peaks in the future.

Furthermore, through a complex process called "prediction" or "prognosis," the Soviets can come close to forecasting how closely a particular athlete will come to reaching his or her career goals, looking ahead many years down the road — and whether the athlete will reach world-class status. This is a complex approach, and as with "modeling," a great number of factors are evaluated, from physical to psychological to so-called medico-biological.

Thus, every facet of athletes and their training is analyzed, and often improvements in their day-to-day work-outs are suggested that will ultimately result in improved performance. This process has become an integral part of the training of Soviet athletes, particularly those who show potential for becoming top competitors.

It is important not to become discouraged by reading how sophisticated sports technology has become in the U.S.S.R. For as I suggest throughout this book, most of the Soviet techniques are adaptable to the American athlete. Those already mentioned in this chapter will be discussed in more depth later. So will breakthroughs like the following, which are all products of years of innovative research:

   *   Scientists in the U.S.S.R. are determining the exact doses of nutrients needed by athletes in particular sports and at specific levels of proficiency. They have also created nutrient drinks ranging from carbohydrate to electrolyte beverages, which are used to help athletes recuperate quickly from competition or rigorous workouts.

   * A training technique called "dynamic isometrics," which incorporates slow movements into the isometric system, has been developed by the Soviets. Adaptations are made for different sports, altering the degree of tensing and relaxing of muscles.

   * Unusual sleds and swings, and a variety of jumping exercises, have been created to help athletes develop explosive leg power.

   * Specially designed pressure chambers are used by Soviet athletes for recuperation and injury rehabilitation. After the athlete places an arm or a leg into the chamber, the atmospheric pressure within the tube is raised or

lowered, stimulating the healing process. Pressure chambers are also used for "baro-oxygenation," in which concentrated oxygen is inhaled to accelerate recovery. Electrical stimulation and sophisticated massage techniques are also used to help the athlete recover from workouts.

* "Auto-conditioning" psychological techniques are routinely used by athletes in training and during competition. Also called "self-regulation" or "autogenic training" autosuggestion helps athletes cope with the tension associated with international meets by teaching them to control and manage their emotional states.

Many of the coaches I know in the West have been initially resistant to trying anything that comes out of the Soviet Union. But once they see techniques like these in action and witness their benefits, they often become much more receptive to what the Soviets have to offer. The Eastern-bloc nations haven't been secretive about what their research laboratories have produced. Almost all of it is available for our use. And as the rest of this book will demonstrate, these techniques may have a positive impact on your own athletic performance.

Chapter 3 Addendum

Since writing this book, I have found myself appreciating Russian sports research even more. To understand this, it is necessary to show the distinction between Russian and American sports research. Also, you should know of the relationships between researchers and coaches prior to the breakup of the Soviet Union and to some extent even now, and the present scene in the U.S.

Most of the major Russian coaching and training methods came from their research and practical experiences based on the research that was done. During the cold war, many of the top coaches were not only former competitive athletes, but many of them were also scientists as for example, Drs. Bondarchuk and Verkhoshansky who are becoming familiar names in the United States. Verkhoshanksky spent most of his time doing research and working with selected track and field athletes, mainly jumpers back in the 1960's and 70's and then later headed up the Sports Research Institute. Practical applications of his works can be found in his book, *Special Strength Training* and in many articles in the *Soviet Sports Review*. See www.dryessis.com for more information.

Dr. Bondarchuk was not only an Olympic performer, but he later coached Olympic and World champions and did extensive research on the transfer of training, periodization and other aspects of training. He established correlations between the most commonly used exercises by the worlds best athletes and the level of performance achieved by these athletes. To date, there is nothing like this research being done in the U.S. or other countries. For anyone interested in more information on the transfer of training in sports, see Bondarchuk's book, *Transfer of Training*, now in English and available at www.dryessis.com.

It should also be noted that in the former USSR there were several outstanding individuals who distinguished themselves with the creation of new methods of training and/or expanding or synthesizing the theory of sports training. These individuals were typically professors and/or researchers. However, they did not simply work at the universities with no contact with high level athletes. They were very much involved with hands-on-training of the athletes and their theories evolved from the training of athletes with the use of different methods. This is a concept that has not been expounded upon in the U.S.

In essence, the Russians developed their methods of training from the work done by the professors and coaches in conjunction with one another. They did not evolve in only one field, or solely from the theories of training or the practical results seen by coaches in the field. There was interaction with scientists/professors who often disagreed in regard to particular theories or methods. For example, I have Russian articles, that were written by coaches who disagree with Verkhoshansky's works and recommendations. As a result, the methods of training were constantly evolving and being improved as time went on. The Physical Culture (coaching) Institutes and training camps in each sport played major roles in this.

Even new concepts such as block training did not evolve only from one individual. Most of the initial work came from coaches of elite athletes in Russia and Germany. At present there are at least three Russians who have contributed to our understanding of the block system of training; Verkhoshansky, Bondarchuk and Issurin. Verkhoshansky wrote about block training back in the 1990's. (See Fitness and Sports Review International); Bondarchuk wrote about it and has been and is a utilizer of block training with his athletes while Issurin has written the most comprehensive book on this subject (Block Periodization). It is now available at www.dryessis.com.

In contrast, in the U.S. there have not been any innovations in training in the last 20-30 years. Most of the new methods seen in the training of U.S. athletes are coming from the Russian methods of past years. The only partial exception to this may be in exercise physiology. This appears to be the area in which most US sports research is done. But even here, we do not see the results of the research being applied to any great extent in the cyclical sports.

It is interesting to note that the Russians believe U.S. coaches are more secretive than Russian coaches in addition to not always employing the most effective training methods. An example is in the development of strength. Most U.S. strength coaches believe in high intensity training where the exercises are done at slow speeds with maximum weights, usually in the 1-3 RM (maximum resistance) range. Some believe it should be 10-12RM while others recommend repetitions at faster speeds.

What is often ignored is the role that each zone of exercise intensity can play in a periodization scheme. According to the Russians, no one method can or should be employed year round for maximum effectiveness. This has been proven many times over and is why periodization is so important in the total concept of training. This is borne out in their research as well as in practical experience. For example, they found that all the weight zones have some benefits. The key is knowing when the particular weights should be used, how long they should be used and by whom they should be used. The Russians believe that 80 to 85% of maximum is optimal for athletes. You develop more strength only when needed, but not year-round, except in the iron sports.

Russian sports research was and is very specific. Usually it deals with one specific aspect of the total skill or game component but related in a specific manner to the total skill or game play. For example, in running there are several studies dealing with the role of the ankle joint in the push-off. From their research about twenty years ago, they came to a conclusion—one that was hard to believe at first since it was against all common understandings—that ankle joint extension was the key force producing action in the push-off in running. It was not knee and/or hip joint extension as is still commonly believed in the U.S.

Russian research, in which there was simultaneous recording of muscle activity (EMG's) with synchronized cinematography, found that at the moment of ground contact there is flexion in the hip joint. Thus, the hamstring and gluteus muscles cannot be contracting at the hip joint to propel the body forward. During ground support, these muscles are stretching, undergoing an eccentric contraction. The same happens in the knee joint. During the actual push-off both the hip and knee joints remain slightly bent (flexed) until ground contact is broken. Because of this and after looking at hundreds of top runners, they could only conclude that the push-off was all in the ankle joint. It was the only joint that could apply force to the ground. For the original studies see back issues of the Soviet Sports Review (later the Fitness and Sports Review International).

In the U.S. this conclusion is contested but there is no research to prove otherwise. Some of the research as for example, the Weyand study that has been popularized in the U.S., the researchers found that ground reaction forces played the major role. There is no questioning the fact that ground reaction forces are a major factor. However, the study concluded that all force was generated during contact and everything else that the athlete did was immaterial. Consequently, technique did not play a role and the ankle joint was not important. Everything was related to how much ground reaction forces could be produced. The research gave no indication of how the general reaction force is generated, what joint actions were involved in generating the ground reaction forces or how they could be increased.

Thus, even though it was sound research, it failed to recognize full running technique and the application of the research was skewed. Thus we see some distinct differences between the research done in the Soviet Union and what is presently done in the U.S. In this regard, I usually give credence to the Russian studies mainly because they have valid substantiation and have proven their worth in training. This is the ultimate test.

Another factor that is important in this regard is that the Russian research uses specific populations for their research. As previously brought out, the Soviets had a system for identifying different levels of athletes, as for example, class 3, class 2, class 1, master of sport and honored master of sport. The latter two are the highest levels and class 3 is the lowest (novice) level but still a bona fide athlete. Each level is categorized by specific levels of achievement. For example a sprinters rank is determined by his best time in a 100 or 200m race. Jumpers by their best distance or height achieved, throwers by how far their best throws were and so on. Thus, depending upon the sport, anytime an athlete's rank is mentioned, you know exactly what level of achievement he is capable of attaining.

When Russian research is done, it is done with a specific class or classes of athlete. Therefore the findings of the research are applicable only to the level(s) specified. The reason for this is that in their research, they found that the exercises and training methods used by higher level athletes are not applicable to the lower levels and vice versa. The effects of training for one level of athlete when used with another level athlete, were often detrimental.

This is very different from the research being done in the U.S. For athletes, physical education (kinesiology) majors or local athletes at a particular university are used. In some cases recreational athletes are used. But, we do not know what level of achievement they are capable of. Even on a Division 1 level, there can be a world of difference between the best universities and some of the worst. In fact, some Division 2 and 3 schools may have better performing athletes than in Division 1. Thus, using such criteria does not always support the conclusions. Compounding the problem is that instead of limiting the findings to the particular population, implications are given that they apply to all levels of athletes. Until we get a system of accurately identifying levels of athletes, the research will have little if any impact on helping coaches—or the athletes.

Much of the sports research in the U.S. can be considered redundant or insignificant because it does not make a contribution to a greater understanding of the topic. There is nothing wrong with the studies themselves, as they are done with excellent protocol, statistics, etc. But because populations are not properly identified in regard to sports proficiency complied with poor topic selection, the results have little impact. Part of the reason for this is that most university professors are not familiar with what is going on in the sports world.

They are not familiar with the training philosophy or methods, the exercises used in different sports, or training periodization. It appears that most students simply come up with a topic that seems to be sound to the professor and are given the green light to go ahead with the research. In many cases, the research can be considered "research for the sake of research", rather than research to learn something new and different or to resolve a particular problem.

Another interesting aspect of Russian research is that Russian coaches had direct access to some of the top researchers in their sport. For example, Dr. Bondarchuk told me that he would call upon professor Donskoi whenever he had a question on the mechanics of the throws. Donskoi was one of their top researchers in biomechanics and was very familiar with the throws and the application of science in the throws. Other high level researcher was Djachkov, perhaps the most brilliant biomechanics researcher in the track and field jumps, especially in regard to technique. These and other high level researchers were highly specialized in particular sports or sports events.

It is rare (if at all possible) to find researchers in the U.S. who are comparable to the Russian researchers in regard to depth of knowledge, understanding of the subject matter and its' practical application in training. This fact should be made public so that hopefully, steps can be taken to remedy this situation. It will go a long way toward improving the level of coaching and the ability to have better athletes and teams, especially on the collegiate and professional levels.

I often think how great it would be, if for example, baseball coaches could call on scientists specializing in this area to determine how they could enable the pitcher to throw faster, or be able to have a more effective pitch, or to produce a .400 level hitter. Or it could be a football coach needing to find out how to enhance his players abilities to become better defensively or offensively, etc. But, this appears to be a long way off since most coaches only deal with strategy and tactics not technique skills. Compounding the issue is that many coaches do not even believe some aspects of skill or game play even when they see it with their own eyes.

For example, I found that the first action that linemen perform on the snap of the ball is to stand up and then move forward to make contact. They do not move forward from the three point stance. When I showed this to the coaches on film, which included play by professional and collegiate teams, they refused to believe that this is what takes place. They maintained that it was still done incorrectly and that they were not about to change their teachings. Thus, with this kind of thinking, it is impossible to have any interaction between coaches and scientists.

Based on what the Russians did, an area that I believe can be improved greatly in the U.S., is biomechanical analyses of the athlete's skill performance. We have excellent technology that is far superior to anything that the Russians had in their prime and probably even today. However, the Russians have one major advantage that we to date do not have, and that is experts capable of doing effective visual biomechanical analyses. Even though we have better technology, most of the analyses relate to descriptions of what a performer does in comparison to another performer. One performer by himself is not analyzed. They produce quantitative data with computers but without answering key questions related to the effectiveness of the key actions or overall performance, the data is of limited value. This becomes even more apparent when no solutions to the problem are presented after describing what takes place.

For example, was the force produced at the optimal time? Can additional force be produced? How is the force produced? (or speed, etc.) Was the sequence of all the joint actions correct? Was the timing good? Were there weaknesses in physical abilities in relation to how the skill was performed? Were actions that could lead to injury during performance determined? What could be done to correct or enhance the finding? These are very important questions that are typically ignored but which are addressed by the Russians.

Thus, I am no longer surprised when I do frame by frame tape analyses of athletes that they express amazement at what they see or learn about what they are doing. Even though they have seen films of themselves before, they were not given an analysis nor did they view themselves frame by frame to see exactly what was occurring in each of the joint actions. In addition, they were not given explanations for their actions. When told how effective or how ineffective each of their actions were and how they could be improved to allow them to become even better, they become even more amazed.

This indicates that even though coaches may do an "analysis", it is not in-depth and usually deals with stance and follow through—not the power phase which determines the success of the action. When suggestions are made for improvement, they typically revolve around the obvious such as, It is necessary to throw harder, have a stronger hip or stronger shoulder turn, faster turnover, or something along these lines. But yet, how changes can be accomplished, which exercises should be done to correct or improve an action, etc. are not covered. Thus the athlete is left on his own in terms of trying to make the necessary changes to make his performance better.

The former Soviets had specialized sports journals in which research was reported, as well as specialized sports journals that included training practices, technique analyses with sequence pictures, coaching advice, specialized exercises and so on. It would be great if we too had such journals in the U.S.

These would be journals that could assist coaches and athletes in terms of how they could improve their performance, i.e. how they could produce or become better players. But, player development or the concept of improving athletic performance through specialized exercises, training, technique analysis, etc. is at best, little known.

It appears that is also impossible to have any of this information appear in major media outlets. If you talk to a sports reporter about doing an article on player development you will quickly find out that they rarely understand what player development is about except in general terms. They take for granted that coaches already do this. They do not realize that their concept of player development is in the area of strategy and tactics, not in improving the physical and technical skills and abilities of the athlete. But, if we had practical and applicable research in this area, and if it was reported in different magazines and papers, the information would be of great value to coaches and athletes and could lead to more and better athletes and athletic programs throughout the U.S.

For example, in baseball there are many baseball "training" centers and youth leagues throughout the country. But there is not a single magazine that deals with improving player performance or even instruction on the latest techniques. Of course, there are books but they are general in nature. The books do not have sequential pictures taken from digital film of skill execution with full explanations of what occurs, when it should occur, why it occurs, how it can be improved, etc.

For a better understanding of this concept, I recommend reading books such as *Build a Better Athlete, Explosive Running, Explosive Basketball Training, Explosive Golf, Explosive Tennis* and *Women's Soccer: Using Science to Improve Speed.* These are the only books that have many pages devoted to technique with sequence pictures taken from digital video tape of different level athletes with biomechanical analyses of what they do, whether the technique is effective, why it is effective, how it can be improved, etc. Compare these books to most any other sports books and you will see the major differences.

In regard to youth leagues that are set up to allow for more players to play the sport, on a organized level, it is necessary to revisit the concept of early specialization in sports. Russian research has found that specializing in only one or two sports in youth is not effective for development of a high level athlete. Instead, youngsters should be involved in many different sports and undergo all-round general training. According to their research this is needed to establish the coordination and other abilities that will enable the athlete to become great in any one sport as he goes into his teenage and adult years. There are a few exceptions to this and usually in sports that require the highest development of technical abilities.

Parents rejoice in their youngsters' accomplishments in the youth leagues which cannot be diminished. For this more and more parents are paying anywhere from 50 to 100 or more dollars per hour to hire trainers to improve the athletic performance of their youngsters. They are paying considerable sums to help their children become great athletes. They know that the coach is not able to do this.

But are they getting their money's worth? The experts being hired include personal trainers in the gyms and former athletes (usually professional) who go into the business of training athletes. As brought out previously, and has been substantiated or by the Russians, former athletes can be qualified to improve athletic performance only if they have also been educated in the science of the sport.

Personal trainers for the most part know little to nothing about sports skills while former athletes may know a little more about sports skills and what it takes to be an athlete. But once again,their knowledge of the fine points or even the basic elements of what it takes to be a good runner, thrower, jumper etc. is still lacking greatly. These and other basic sports skills are very complex. This is why just having the athlete run more, or throw more, or jump more (as is commonly done on sports teams) is a poor way —really the slowest way – to improve performance.

Even though youngsters may have great success in the early ages of 9-14, Russian research has shown that most do not have the same enthusiasm or desire to keep playing the sport when they are 16-18! Most of them will drop out. In addition, studies have shown that very few ever make it to the highest levels. The same results are being seen in the United States. This appears to be a fairly universal truth.

Thus, specializing at a very early age is not the answer to becoming a great athlete. The answer lies in training and developing the youngster's potential. This is something that is overlooked in the U.S. but was not in the former Soviet system. The Russians believe that the early years are formative years and much attention should be paid to development of basic technical and physical skills— something that early specialization does not allow. Youngsters are not able to develop the abilities needed to become great at a later age. Understand that the many physical abilities that are needed to be successful are not developed by only playing the sport. Other activities (trainings) are needed to develop these abilities which can then be incorporated into the main sport.

When discussing specialization it is necessary to distinguish general physical preparation (GPP) from specialized physical preparation (SPP). According to the

Russians, in GPP you do many different sports, exercises, etc. that do not always have a direct influence on sports performance. They may however, influence skills or physical qualities as for example, developing greater endurance which allows the athlete to perform better or longer. GPP however, is the type of training most often encountered in the training of U.S. athletes both in the early years as well as in the adult years—even on the professional sports level!

The SPP that was developed by coaches and researchers is one of the cornerstones of the Russian system of training. However, the term specialized has very distinct criteria. Foremost is that the exercise must duplicate the neuromuscular pathway seen in execution of the competitive skill. This means that you must duplicate a portion or portions of the total skill. Also, the exercise must develop strength in the same range of motion as seen in execution of the competitive skill and the exercise must use the same type of muscular contraction as seen in execution of the competitive skill. In some sports the exercise must involve the same energy systems as in the competitive skill. There are still others but these should be sufficient to show how specialized exercises differ from general exercises.

According to the Russians, specialized exercises are most important in the pre-competitive period. The Russians almost exclusively use specialized exercises during this period. In contrast, in the U.S., many athletes are only just getting into shape with general exercises which are continued throughout the season. The concept of such specialized training still has not permeated major sports. But, developing this practice can improve player abilities tremendously on all levels of performance.

There are many more aspects of Russian training that have come from a combination of research and practical experience. Coaches, especially those with a great amount of experience have come up with many new and different methods of training. Some are original, some are in conjunction with researchers, others are modifications of methods developed by other coaches or combinations of these factors.

Some of the methods developed include conjugate and complex training, the stage-complex method, stage-variational method, stage-complex-variational method, stage-variational-complex method, block method, block-complex method, block-complex-variational method, variational method and complex-variational method. These different methods are used at specific times with specific athletes.

According to Bondarchuk, the training method or program selected often depends on the way the athlete responds to the training. For example, some athletes show a rapid increase in improvement and then a gradual leveling off and sometimes even a decrease at the end of a training period—a specific period of sports form development. Other athletes are very slow to show gains initially but show rapid progress at the end of the training cycle while still others show steady gains throughout the cycle. Thus, the selection of methods used, when they are used in the periodization scheme and with which athlete, depends on the characteristics and needs of the athlete. As can be seen, it is a very sophisticated and individualized process.

Other methods that have been derived from research and/or from practical experience are explained in more detail in the speed-strength and innovations chapters. More information can also be found in *Transfer of Training* by Anatoly Bondarchuk, and *Block Periodization* by Vladimir Issurin.

Chapter 4:

THE NEWEST TRAINING INNOVATIONS: How They Can Help You

When I was studying for my Ph.D. in physical education at the University of Southern California in the late 1950s and early 1960s, some of my peers frequently asked me, "Why is the U.S.S.R. so successful in sports?" Even though the Soviets had participated in international meets for barely a decade at that time, they had already established themselves as a major athletic power, demonstrating superiority in events ranging from distance running to the high jump to weightlifting to gymnastics. At the 1956 and 1960 Olympics, their women athletes in particular were outstanding, consistently outshining their Western counterparts.

Because both my parents were born in Russia, emigrating to the U.S. early in this century, my fellow students assumed I might have some insights into why the Soviet athletes excelled so often. But I had no answers for them then, although I was becoming increasingly curious myself about the success of the Eastern-bloc competitors.

As a result, I began spending time in the library, searching for information about the sports training techniques used in the socialist countries. I discovered that the Library of Congress regularly received several Russian-language sports publications from the U.S.S.R., and I started reading them.

While these journals concentrated on sports, they were highly scientific, and I was frequently forced to look up the definitions of technical terms in my Russian dictionary, even though my proficiency in the language was reasonably good, it was a laborious process. But as I proceeded, I became increasingly intrigued by what I was learning. It was clear that the U.S.S.R. was years, even decades, ahead of the West in its understanding and training of athletes.

In subsequent years, as I studied the Soviet system further and met with Eastern-bloc coaches both in the U.S. and in their own countries, I continued to be amazed at their knowledge and expertise. For instance, during one of my first meetings with coaches from the U.S.S.R., we were discussing some of the fine points of the hammer throw and how centrifugal forces influenced this event. One of them turned to me and said, "You personally know a lot about biomechanics, so I'm sure you understand all that we're saying here." I was too embarrassed to tell him that though I was familiar with what Western researchers had discovered about biomechanics [technique analysis], his own expertise was far ahead of mine.

Fortunately, many of the breakthroughs that have occurred in the Soviet sports labs can be utilized by athletes here. In this chapter, I will introduce you to some of the newer sports concepts that have been developed in the U.S.S.R., most of which are unknown in the United States. I will also show you how these techniques can be incorporated into your own training schedule. No matter what role fitness and sports play in your life, you can benefit from these Soviet innovations.

PERIODIZATION

Several years ago, the U.S.S.R. national volleyball team came to America to play our national team. One afternoon in San Diego, after a rigorous match between the two teams the night before, the Soviet coach asked for a large outdoor field that his athletes could use.

Once we had set them up at a nearby park—-just hours before their next match with the U.S. team—the Soviet volleyball players jogged at a leisurely pace for about a mile. Then they marked off boundaries for a full-length soccer field, and began playing an all-out, strenuous game of soccer. Dozens of times over the next half hour, the athletes ran from one end of the field to the other, playing energetically until their coach blew his whistle, seemingly bringing the afternoon workout to a halt.

But they weren't finished yet—not by a long shot. The coach lined up his players, and for the next ten minutes, he led them through a series of deep jumps; squat jumps, lunges, major hops. Then he grabbed the soccer ball again and announced, "Okay, let's change sides!" The soccer game resumed.

For another thirty minutes the athletes played vigorously, without a single time-out to catch their breath. A television news crew had come by, and, impressed by the skill and endurance of the players, asked me, "What soccer team is this?" To their surprise, I responded, "They're not soccer players. They're the Soviet *volleyball* team." That night, incidentally, the athletes from the U.S.S.R. defeated the American team in three straight volleyball games.

94

More than anything else, I came away from that experience marveling at how finely conditioned the Soviets were. They not only played outstanding volleyball, but their high-level training had given them amazing versatility and all-around skills. To them, a spirited soccer game at full throttle was fun and recreation, as well as a "warm-up" for volleyball competition that night.

A major reason for the excellent conditioning of athletes in the U.S.S.R. is the unique way in which their training program is structured. Under their "periodization" system, each athlete's yearly conditioning plan is broken down into four distinct stages: the general preparatory period, the specialized preparatory period, the competitive period, and the transitional or postcompetitive period. From one stage to the next, the athlete works in a progressive manner, changing his training regimen as he goes along.

The results of periodization speak for themselves. Not only do Soviet athletes excel in their own sports, but they are also in excellent all-around shape. Even in defeat, it is clear that they have been superbly prepared and conditioned.

Periodization (or "cycling") is not a new idea in the U.S.S.R., even though it is barely known and rarely practiced outside the Eastern bloc. Its origins date back two to three decades, when Soviet research first demonstrated that high-level athletes could best be developed by placing them on a well-organized, systematic schedule. Very young athletes— still five, ten, or even fifteen years away from Olympic-level competition—are placed on a multiyear program aimed at bringing out their optimum potential. (It has been calculated, for example, that it takes between nine and twelve years to develop a top volleyball player, who will peak between the ages of twenty-three and twenty-seven.)

Each year of this lengthy training saga is then "periodized" into monthly and sometimes weekly cycles, incorporating the four stages mentioned above. The length of each period is adjusted for each athlete, depending on his or her level of physical preparation, mastery of the sport, competitive schedule, and other factors. For instance, if there are two major periods of competition during the year (e.g., an indoor and an outdoor track-and-field season), the athlete's schedule will be broken down so he or she goes through the complete four-period cycle twice. At times a particular period will last for only a few weeks, but none is ever eliminated completely. This is what occurs in each of the four stages of training:

GENERAL PREPARATORY PERIOD

The Soviets believe that unless an athlete's general fitness base is excellent, he or she will achieve little success in sports. So in this initial phase of the cycle, athletes aim primarily at getting into shape and forming a foundation for the training to come. They actually spend only a limited amount of time playing their particular sport — usually no more than 20 percent of the training schedule unless they have a real need for additional skill development. Instead, they strive for all-around physical fitness. Thus, about 80 percent of their workout is devoted to overall conditioning of the body — all major joints, muscles, ligaments, and other support structures — with special attention paid to areas of bodily weakness.

Volume is the key during this period. The emphasis is on many different kinds of exercises for all the joints of the body, Movements that require twisting, bending, leaning, and swinging are part of the schedule, and dumbbells and barbells are often used. At the same time, young (teenage) athletes continue to improve basic skills such as running, throwing, jumping, and hitting. Slow long-distance running at a specific heart rate (140 to 160 beats per minute for top-level athletes) is also emphasized to build up cardiorespiratory and aerobic fitness.

During this time, the Soviets also emphasize strength training. Research demonstrates that, more than any other single factor, strength helps prevent injuries. For example, if a football player steps into a divot as he's running down the field, his muscles will instinctively contract to minimize excessive movement that can cause serious damage. However, if training hasn't made his muscles strong enough, then his tendons will have to take the brunt of the force, and if they fail, then the ligaments must assume this role. The muscles and tendons are elastic and designed to stretch, but that isn't the case with ligaments. If they become stretched, the athlete may find himself in need of surgery to repair them. It's an injury that proper strength training could have prevented.

To build up strength during the general preparatory period, Soviet athletes spend a lot of time in the weight room. On the days between strength workouts, many general developmental exercises with high repetitions are used. This is needed to strengthen the joints, and especially the tendons and ligaments.

Based on Soviet research, here is what I recommend to achieve maximum all-around strength. Athletes should divide the body into three parts—upper, midsection, and lower—and perform exercises that concentrate on each of these regions. For instance, you can choose from the following exercises to develop each of the bodily areas:

Upper Body:

bench presses
lat pulldowns
overhead presses
biceps curls
head circles
push-ups
bar dips
triceps kickbacks
wrist curls
dumbbell flyes
concentration curls
cable crossovers

front arm raises
lateral arm raises
arm circles
triceps extensions
pull-ups
incline and decline presses
supination-pronation
reverse flyes
behind-the-neck presses
ulna and radial flexions
upright, seated, and reverse wrist curls bent-over rows

Midsection:

sit-ups
back raises
back raises with a twist
reverse trunk twists
crunches

bench sit-ups
side bends

sit-ups with a twist
hanging leg raises
sit-ups on a glute-ham developer
floor side bends
Russian twists (horizontal shoulder rotations)
reverse sit-ups

Lower Body:

toe raises
leg presses
hip-joint extensions
dead lifts
leg squats
lunges
heel raises

squats
knee curls
walking lunges
glute-ham-gastroc raises
hip-joint flexions and abductions
good mornings

Ideally, the general preparatory period should last at least three months (though the range is from one to four months), with a gradual transition into the next period (specialized preparatory training). Thus, if three months are allowed for general training, specialized exercises are introduced in growing numbers in the final month. Likewise, in the first month of the specialized period, there is a continuation of some of the general preparatory training. After three months dedicated solely to getting into shape, is it any wonder that the Soviet athletes are in such excellent physical condition?

SPECIALIZED PREPARATORY PERIOD

In the next period, some generalized conditioning continues to take place, but most of the athlete's workout schedule—about 80 percent—shifts gears. Training becomes selective, with an extremely high correlation to the athlete's specific sport. At this time, the volume of work—that is, the actual number of exercises and repetitions performed—decreases, but the intensity and complexity of the workouts increase.

This is a very demanding period in the training cycle. Athletes will be doing maximum work, drawing upon all of their body's capacity. In the weight room, they may increase the amount of pounds they handle, the speed with which exercises are performed, or both speed and strength simultaneously. Without the base developed during the general preparatory period, many athletes would fall by the wayside during this time.

Let me give you an example. Though American football does not exist in the U.S.S.R., here is how the program could be adapted to football players in the U.S. They would concentrate on exercises specific to play action during this period— that is, those with movements that duplicate the motions they go through during an actual game. For instance, they might do leg squats with fast upward motion, jumps out of a squat, split squat jumps, walk-leap lunges, and bench step-ups with the thigh parallel to the ground to develop strength and power and to simulate starting leg action. Or they would focus upon continuous pulls, which include a dead lift, followed by an upright row and then a heel raise. Or they might perform several "good mornings" (bending forward from the hips with a barbell on the shoulders), followed by squats and overhead presses.

For more explosiveness, football players would concentrate on depth jumps, as well as arm depth jumps and hand jumps over objects. To practice repelling an opponent, they would do push-up jumps with a clap, side jumps, and a springy "wheelbarrow walk" on the hands while their legs are held by a partner. Or they would practice throwing a shot or medicine ball using two hands in front of the chest. Quarterbacks would do exercises to improve their throwing, such as medial rotation with the hand dropped low behind the head; for explosiveness, they would perform overhead, three-quarter sidearm, and full sidearm medicine-ball catches and throws.

Specific agility exercises would also be incorporated into the program. The football player might perform open-field exercises such as jumping over pits and bushes, followed by forward or side rolls. He could also practice a particular skill under unusual conditions—perhaps starting and running on sandy ground, or throwing passes with and against the wind. Leg (hip) abductions would be used to improve side moves, along with forward and side jumps and maze runs.

Flexibility exercises are also utilized during this period. Though flexibility will be discussed in depth later in this chapter, it also belongs in a discussion of the football player's training program. Because football is such a physical sport, the athlete should be merging vigorously performed (dynamic) flexibility exercises with strength training to minimize susceptibility to injury.

Specialized training lasts from one to four months. During this time, intensity increases greatly as volume declines. Near or at the end of this period, the athlete will be in top form. He'll be ready for competition.

Actually, if he has trained sufficiently during these preparatory periods, the athlete should be ready—and able—to compete at a higher level than ever before, even though his longevity as a competitor has increased by another year. Soviet athletes such as triple-jumper V. Saneev, for instance, have participated in a remarkable four Olympic Games, performing at peak, medal-winning levels each time. Saneev's preparation has paid off handsomely again and again.

COMPETITIVE PERIOD

Some elements of competition have already been present in the general and specialized preparatory periods, with team mates vying with one another to see who can kick farthest; throw hardest, or run fastest. Finally, however, the true test of months of training arrives. The athlete should now be peaking just as the competitive season begins.

In the U.S.S.R., the competitive period is usually subdivided into two stages: the early competitive (one to two months) and the main competitive period (one to four months depending on the sport). In the first stage, the athletes are not yet striving for maximum performances, but are merely adjusting to the competitive environment. In the latter stage however, they are attempting to achieve the best performances of which they are capable. There is rarely any holding back for another meet—or another year.

No matter at what plateau athletes may find themselves however, they rarely attempt to improve their physical strength or level of fitness during the competitive season, particularly if they are part of a team sport. Instead, they channel most of their attention toward refining their technique in their specific sport, as well as learning more about strategy and tactics.

For basketball players, for instance, shooting is a precise act, and if they were to become stronger in mid-season, it could undermine their shooting "touch." So during the season, they really don't want to become stronger (or weaker, for that matter). As a result, players spend the competitive period working on team play and perfecting new offenses and defenses, while maintaining their present strength levels.

Athletes in the individual sports may continue working to make themselves stronger—like the weightlifter and the shot-putter, who are constantly striving to increase their strength and speed-strength capabilities. But as they continue building up their strength, following a precise training schedule, they are working on technique as well while a football lineman or a baseball outfielder could also join those who are increasing their strength during the competitive period, the quarterback or pitcher would run the risk of disrupting his throwing technique by doing so.

TRANSITIONAL PERIOD

The athlete who may have ridden the bench during the competitive period will not need time for recuperation afterward. Not having endured the physical and emotional stress of competition, he or she is able to continue on with regular training sessions, just as before. This athlete is not burned out.

But those who have competed must move into a transitional period of so-called active rest. Following months of rigorous games or meets, they need a break from their sport and the stresses they have endured. As one Soviet researcher has written, the purpose of this period "is to prevent an ever-increasing cumulative effect of training and competition so that the athlete does not go into a state of overtraining." In short, it's a well-earned and necessary breathing spell.

The athlete who has just gone through high-intensity competition may also need some time for rehabilitation—healing those minor injuries that may have nagged at him or her all season long. The transitional period, then, is a time for physical healing as well.

During this phase, however, the athlete does not sit idly by, wasting precious time that could be put to some use in the overall training program. The mind may take a break, but except in the case of injuries, the body remains active, and other sports become important. The athlete participates in sports different from the chosen specialty—which provide a change of pace but still a chance to keep strong.

The Soviets believe that while playing other sports, the central nervous system is permitted to relax and "unwind" from the tremendous strain it experienced during competition. The mind is allowed to concentrate on something different, and other nervous pathways and reflexes are used.

So the volleyball player may play basketball or handball; the long-distance runner might still do some running in the postcompetitive period, but it will be mostly "fun" running.

A change of environment may also be helpful during this time. If you've been living and training in the city, you may benefit from several weeks in the mountains or at the seashore, perhaps swimming, hiking or climbing. This is a way to recharge emotional batteries and ensure that attitudes will be positive once the new training cycle begins again.

The transitional period is not particularly long—usually twenty to thirty days. Once it is completed, athletes embark on the next yearly training cycle, and because they have not neglected themselves physically during the transition, they begin the new cycle at the level they had achieved at the end of the previous year. Thus, the strength, speed, agility, and flexibility they had gained are retained from the end of one training year to the beginning of the next. However, because of the transitional period, they are fully rested, healed, and have recuperated from competition. They are ready to start again.

PERIODIZATION IN THE U.S.?

At the university where I teach, I recently instituted a new class in the physical education department on specialized preparatory training and exercises. But when I first proposed the idea for such a class, many of my colleagues reacted skeptically. In fact, many did not know what I was talking about. The concept of periodization was completely unknown to them.

Most athletes here have not heard of periodization either, and thus have not yet begun to use it in their training program. If you're a recreational runner or swimmer, for example, you probably follow the same training regimen each time you train, without any variation as you move through the year. And if you're competing on the high school or college level, the situation is even worse. There are clear obstacles that prevent periodization from being implemented, even if there is some interest among your coaches in doing so.

NCAA regulations, as well as those on the high school level, allow teams only a short preseason in which to get in shape before competition begins. In most cases, it lasts no more than two to six weeks before the first game or match Can you get someone into shape in just two weeks? In the U.S.S.R., the question itself would be considered ridiculous. After all, athletes there are accustomed to many months of organized training before competition.

It is true that American athletes can train on their own in the weeks and months before formal workouts begin. But how many really do? It takes formidable dedication to train on your own, and not many will. Working out can be a hard, miserable experience.

I remember despising training myself, complaining, "Not again today; I'm going to get all beat up out there." Even the most organized workouts are not something you look forward to. You do it because you're looking ahead to the day of competition. That's what you love. But you're a rare breed if you practice on your own. When the coach isn't standing over them, most athletes do little or nothing to get or stay in shape.

Looking back to my own athletic career, however, I can now see how much better I could have been if I had known about periodization. When I was competing, we had only a few weeks to get into shape, and then were thrust into the season I never got into top shape until the *end of* the season.

Because the competition for college scholarships and pro contracts is so much stiffer today, some U.S. athletes are beginning to recognize that their training should be placed on £ year-round schedule, though most are training just as American athletes did a generation ago. I am convinced that our athletes could be better prepared with periodization— whether they are formally competing or merely running 1 (kilometer races for enjoyment. If you run marathons, for instance, your times would probably improve by dividing you] training schedule into four distinct periods centered on the one or two key marathons you run each year.

Here is how this might work. When I help marathon runners create their training schedules, I suggest primarily aerobic endurance workouts in the general preparatory period. That means low-intensity, volume running—a lot of running— and running over great distances, generally at below-maximum speeds. During these runs, the heart rate should stabilize at about 140 to 160 beats per minute for the serious marathoner whose aim is to win the event.

In this same period, I also suggest some strength work in the weight room. It should involve not just the legs but the total body. As the marathoner learns in his or her first 26-mile run, the entire body is involved in the event. Thus, I recommend some weight training for the biceps in order to help keep the forearms at a 90-degree angle to the upper arms, a: the upper arms move forward and back throughout the race It is also important to work on the shoulders and the back and abdominal muscles, whose strength can keep the pelvic girdle from rotating excessively over the 26 miles, as well as maintaining an upright posture during the run.

As strength is built up, however, technique must not be ignored. For instance, as they run, athletes should concentrate on landing first on the balls of their feet, not on their heels, a: is typically advocated. Why? As you land on the heel, with your lead leg far out in front of the rest of your body, it is like putting on the brakes. The entire body is jarred — through the ankle, knee, hip, and back. Shoe manufacturers attempt to compensate for this by putting well-cushioned, built-up heels on their shoes. But when the heel on the shoe begins to wear down, problems intensify and injuries develop. Thus, during the generalized preparatory period, the Soviets have their runners work extensively on proper running technique.

Once marathoners shift to the specialized preparatory period, they begin alternating slow, distance jogging with periods of faster running. I often suggest *the fartlek* (or speed-play) technique, which mixes bursts of speed — sprints of 100 to 300 yards — with longer periods (five to ten minutes) of the usual more moderate pace.

Some background on the demands of running are in order here: When you run at a fast pace (a heart rate exceeding 160 beats per minute*), your aerobic or oxygen system often cannot keep up with your energy demands. As you reach and pass this threshold, your energy needs must be met by a mixed energy system of aerobics and anaerobics (without oxygen), This anaerobic component calls upon fats stored within the body for energy. If your energy requirements continue to grow (heart rate over 180 beats per minute), then this mix of aerobic-anaerobic systems may not be enough, and you will have to rely exclusively on your anaerobic system. On race day, in fact, you'll call upon this anaerobic system alone for your finishing kick. While aerobic running will provide staying power, anaerobic running will provide the explosive sprint at the end of the race.

If you run middle distances, say 10 kilometers, you should devote more of your training time to pure anaerobic work — that is, there should be more of an emphasis on sprints and fast running. While marathoners should be spending 4 to 5 percent of their workout time running at high speeds, the 10-kilometer runner should raise that figure to 6 to 10 percent.

The Soviets have found that for the marathon, the key to success is to run as long and as fast as possible using only aerobic energy, hovering on the brink of the mixed aerobic- anaerobic phase.

* Heart rates will vary depending on the age and level of fitness of the individual.

So before you slip into the combination phase at a heart rate of 160 beats a minute, for example, you ideally should be running at a rate of 159 to achieve maximum efficiency. If you can run with this kind of economy, you'll use less energy, and thus have more left to draw upon when you really have to increase your speed—as in the final kick.

However, there may soon be some changes made in the way we train aerobically. During my visit to the U.S.S.R. in 1986, I learned about new research showing that it's possible to produce a true aerobic effect while doing strength training. Thus, rather than putting in additional mileage to develop aerobic capabilities, you can mix in some strength training instead.

The Soviets believe that this new approach will cut down on injuries, since in pure aerobic training, the heart, circulatory, and respiratory systems tend to develop at a faster rate than general strength. This leaves the athlete susceptible to injuries, which will probably be avoidable as strength training is emphasized.

Although this new aerobic strength program is still being refined, it works something like this: An amount of weight to be lifted is chosen so that in eight to ten seconds the athlete can execute eight to twelve repetitions of a particular exercise, such as the squat. A total of five to six sets is performed, with a rest period of sixty seconds between sets. Over time, the number of sets is increased to ten to twelve, and the rest periods are decreased to ten to thirty seconds each.

New approaches to training such as this will ultimately be integrated into the periodization program in the U.S.S.R., which is central to the entire training philosophy there. As I mentioned earlier, not only do the Soviets now split up each year into periods, but they also divide each athlete's entire career into four distinct phases that carry the same names— the general preparatory, specialized preparatory, competitive, and transitional periods. In this multiyear system, pre-adolescents would first be put through several years of preliminary (or general preparatory) training, in which the aim is to become an all-around, versatile athlete. All their physical qualities—strength, endurance, agility, flexibility—are worked on at this time. They do take some specialized training as well, but 80 percent of the training would be devoted to getting into shape.

After three to four years, typically beginning at ages fourteen or fifteen, the youngster begins to specialize in a sport. Perhaps 80 percent of his or her time would be devoted to that sport, while the remainder is spent on general conditioning.

As athletes enter their prime—perhaps at age seventeen or eighteen (depending on the sport)—they then move into the competitive phase of their careers. They join the Soviet national teams and compete in international events, or if their talents aren't up to this standard, they compete on sports-club teams (analogous to professional teams in the U.S.). In this period, they actually move through two phases—intensive, deep training, followed by several years designed to further improve their performance, (See Table 8 for the multiyear training of a short-distance runner.)

Finally, once they are no longer able to compete, they go through a transitional period or "withdrawal" from heavy training. They still work out for a year or two, but do so on a much lighter scale that eases them out of the physical and emotional strain of so many years of intense training.

No matter what sport you enjoy or compete in, you should consider adapting some form of periodization into your training. Its principles have been researched and tested over the past twenty to thirty years. Nearly every

American athlete, I believe, could come closer to his or her own maximum achievement by dividing the workout schedule into four distinct periods.

TABLE 8 Model for multiyear training of short-distance runner (Per Prof. V.P. Filin)						
Stage	Age (yrs)	Basic Task of training	Basic Method of training	Basic means of training	Allowable Training loads (competitive period)	Approximate level of developments of the main physical qualities
Preliminary Preparation	10-13	1-All around physical preparation 2-Mastery of running technique and other sports exercises 3-Developmet of speed in all forms	1-Play 2-Repetitive 3-Mixed	1-Movement and sports games 2-Running short distances 3-Jumps and jumping exercises 4-Throwing	1-Sports or movement games—30min 2-Repeat running for 30 min (5-7 times) 3-Repeat runs for 80 min (3-4 times)	SPEED 1-Tempo in running 20m with a running start: 2.5-4.8 strides 2-60m run, 7.7-7.8sec SPEED-STRENGTH QUALITIES 1-Long jump from place, 240-245cm 2-Triple jump from place, 740-760cm
Beginning Specialization	14-16	1-All around physical preparation 2-Mastery of running technique and other track and field exercises 3-Developmet of speed-strength qualities 4-Development of general endurance	1-Play 2-Repetitive 3-Circuit 4-Mixed	1-Sports games 2-Running short distances 3-Specialized preparatory exercises 4-Exercises with small weights 5-Jumps and jump exercises 6-Throwing	1-Running with a start, 6-8 runs, 30-40 meters each 2-Repeat running, 3-4 runs, 60-80 meters each 3-Repeat running, 2-3 runs, 150 meters each 4-Specialized preparatory exercises, 6-8, 80 meters each 5-Exercises with the barbell (50-75% of body weight). 5-6 sets 6-Cross-country running, 15-20 min	SPEED 1-60 m run, 7.2-7.3 sec SPEED-STRENGTH QUALITIES 1-Long jump from place, 235-250 cm 2-Triple jump from place, 820-840 cm

110

Deep training in the chosen event	17-18	1-Development of specialized physical qualities of the sprinter (speed, speed-strength qualities, specialized endurance) 2-Improvement in sprint technique 3-Acquiring competitive experience	1-Repeat 2-Circuit 3-Mixed 4-Competitive	1-Running short distances 2-Specialized preparatory exercises with weights 3-Specialized preparatory exercises 4-Jumps and jumping exercises 5-Throwing	1-Running with a start, 8-10 runs, 30-40 meters each 2-Repeat runs, 3-4 runs, 80-100 meters each 3-Repeat runs, 2-3 runs, 150-200 meters each 4- Specialized preparatory exercises, 8-10, 80 meters each 5- Barbell exercises (50-75% of body weight) 6-8 sets	SPEED 1-60m run-6 8-9 sec SPEED-STRENGTH QUALITIES 1-Long jump from place, 290-310 cm 2-Triple jump from place, 820-840 cm
Sports improvement	19 and older	1-Development of specialized physical qualities of the sprinter 2- Improvement in sprint technique 3-Acquiring competitive experience	1-Repeat 2-Circuit 3-Mixed 4-Competitive	1-Running short distances 2-Specialized preparatory exercises 3-Exercises with weights 4-Jumps and jumping exercises 5-Throwing	1-Running with a start, 10-12 runs, 30-50 meters each 2-Repeat runs, 4-5 runs, 80-100 meters each 3-Repeat runs, 3-4 runs, 150-200 meters each 4- Specialized preparatory exercises, 10-12, 80-100 meters each	SPEED 1-60m run-6.6-6.7 sec SPEED-STRENGTH QUALITIES 1-Long jump from place, 310-320 cm 2-Triple jump from place, 880-900 cm

FLEXIBILITY

Flexibility refers to the range of motion of a joint. In simple terms, it is a measure of how far you can move your arms, legs, and trunk around each joint. If your sport calls for reaching and bending—and that includes swimming, long jumping, volleyball, basketball, gymnastics, and others—then you need flexibility in order to excel.

In the U.S., many coaches are convinced that the more flexible you are, the better. Consequently, you can hardly climb out of bed in the morning without being told to stretch. Stretch before you run. Stretch before you lift. Stretch *after* you run or lift. And then stretch some more. It's virtually a cliché.

But is all that stretching really necessary? Maybe not, particularly to the degree that many American coaches promote it. In the U.S.S.R., researchers have now concluded that for most sports you need not be as flexible as athletes like Olga Korbut. Yes, increased flexibility will help prevent injuries, but only to a certain extent. The ability to place your foot behind your head has few practical (or injury-preventing) applications if you're a cyclist, or if you play tennis or baseball.

Obviously, flexibility has an important place in most training programs, with the goal being to gain enough suppleness to execute the movements required in your sport. Keep in mind, however, that to a large extent your flexibility is determined by your genes. Your muscles, tendons, and ligaments can stretch only so far and no farther. There are some anatomical limitations as well, with certain joints permitting more range of motion than others. The shoulder is a ball-and-socket joint and permits movement in all directions; the elbow is a hinge joint and allows only flexion and extension.

Most people, however, do not fully utilize their potential for flexibility. As you become more flexible, you are stretching your muscles and tissue, literally making them longer and looser. That, in turn, increases their range of motion, making moves possible in your sport without any pulling or tearing.

But too much flexibility by itself can backfire. Some Soviet research has shown that flexibility exercises initially stretch the muscles and their connective tissues. Once they have been stretched to their limits, however, the only way to achieve

112

even more flexibility is by stretching the ligaments, which, as we have noted, don't have the elasticity of the muscles and tendons. Thus, when the ligaments are stretched, they remain stretched. As this happens, the joints they hold together will weaken, making you *more* susceptible to injury.

Luckily, there is a way to avoid injuries that occur in this way. The Soviets have now developed a system in which flexibility exercises are combined with the strength training I've already discussed. Whenever an athlete is doing a lot of stretching, he or she is also instructed to do strength work to make the muscles stronger, which in turn holds the joints firmly together.

In the U.S. we do nothing like this. Coaches here emphasize so-called passive or static stretching, even overstretching, with no strength exercises to complement them. Whether or not you know the terms, you've probably done a lot of it yourself. It involves slow, sustained, and controlled stretching, in which the muscle is lengthened and then held in the final position for several seconds.

For athletes in certain sports, static stretching makes sense. For instance, swimmers in the Soviet Union who are trying to develop more ankle-joint flexibility will concentrate on static stretching exercises.

It is important to feel a stretch in the muscle. But if you feel pain, you've gone too far. Also, if you're having a teammate hold or push you further into your stretch, you're asking for even more trouble.

Many times, I've seen football coaches put their players through a stretch that makes me cringe just to watch it. The athletes get down on their knees, sit back upon their feet, and then a teammate stands in front of them and pushes their chest as far back as possible. True, the knee gets stretched, but it often also gets overstretched and actually weakens. In football, where the knee is so vulnerable anyway, it is foolish to subject players to an exercise that actually makes them *more* prone to injury.

In much the same way, American basketball players are often guided through a standing stretch that is commonly used by runners as well. Leaning against a wall with their right hand, they reach behind with their left hand and grab the toes of their left foot. Then they gently pull their heel toward their buttocks and hold for a few seconds. But in basketball, or running, how often do you bend the knee like that? It never happens. And as the Soviets have learned, flexibility for flexibility's sake may do more harm than good.

Most injuries occur at the extremes in the range of motion —for example, at the rotator cuff as the pitcher rears his arm way back—so the athlete does need some flexibility work. But while Soviet athletes do a certain amount of static stretching, it is always only slightly beyond the range of motion required by their sport, and it is always accompanied by strength training.

I really can't stress too much the importance of this strength aspect of flexibility training. Several years ago, a skier came to me for advice after having been diagnosed as having stretched ligaments in both shoulders. Whenever he planted a pole to make a quick turn, his shoulder would dislocate. Doctors had recommended surgery to shorten the overstretched ligaments.

I had a different suggestion. I advised that before he submitted to the surgeon's scalpel, he try a weight-training program designed to develop the shoulder-joint muscles. He agreed and gradually built up strength in this region. Six months later he was able to resume ski racing, without having to undergo surgery. He has continued to do the exercises and has never again experienced a dislocated shoulder.

As Soviet athletes move closer to the competitive period, they tend to shift from static stretching to so-called dynamic stretching, which involves bouncing or other movement to achieve a stretching effect. The contrast is apparent at international track-and-field meets; while Western athletes are doing a lot of slow, static stretches during their warmups, the Soviets and the East Germans are bouncing and jumping in order to achieve a stronger stretch and to improve muscle resiliency. Though American coaches have become afraid of bobbing movements for fear of causing injuries, the Soviet athletes are so finely tuned (because of their strength and speed-strength training techniques) that they can do dynamic work without risking any damage.

Again, the Soviet athletes go *slightly* beyond the range of motion they need in their sport, thus providing a little reserve if they should deviate from their normal movements during training or competition. It's a safety valve that can help prevent injuries.

The Soviets continue to refine certain exercises that have both stretching and strength-enhancing properties. Here's one of the more popular, commonly known as dumbbell flyes: Lie on your back on a narrow exercise bench, with the arms extended straight above the chest, and dumbbells in your hands. Then lower the arms slowly to the side, below the level of the bench. As you move the arms down, there will be a tremendous stretch across the front part of the chest.

Once you've reached the bottom of your range of motion, begin raising the dumbbells. As you elevate them, the exercise changes from a stretching to a strength maneuver. Particularly in those first few inches that the weights are raised, the new range of motion is being strengthened.

While most athletes can benefit from exercises like this, perhaps none need a full range of flexibility more than gymnasts. In fact, because gymnasts need such finely tuned flexibility (along with strength) in their sport, other athletes often look to them for training ideas. A growing number of Soviet athletes are now working on their own flexibility in the gymnastics room. Some are touching their toes to their hands while hanging from a high bar. Or they are performing various movements on the gymnastics horse to work on hip-joint flexibility. Some are even joining aerobic-dancing classes, which involve many dynamic flexibility and strength movements.

Not long ago I observed a Soviet gymnast perform an exercise that still makes me shudder each time I think about it. He was holding a heavy dumbbell in each hand, and had placed his feet on two blocks that were more than a meter apart. Then he started to lower himself into the splits, ultimately going past the point where his legs were parallel to the ground. His buttocks were soon *below* the level of the blocks. Ouch!

After a momentary pause, the gymnast then began raising himself back into an upright position, working against the resistance that the dumbbells provided. As he did, particularly in those first few seconds of movement, he was building strength in this new range of motion that his body had just entered. So not only had he improved his flexibility, but he was also enhancing strength in the area to minimize the risk of injury.

One final note about what the Soviets have discovered about flexibility. If you're a runner, you've probably been told that ten minutes of stretching exercises are absolutely essential before you begin your jog. And most runners have taken the advice seriously—leaning against telephone poles or placing their legs up on a hurdle to stretch before they start running.

In the majority of cases, however, these joggers may be wasting their time. While it's true that a high-level, competitive runner should certainly perform some stretches before he or she hits the track, the average recreational runner—

who may jog three or four miles several times a week to stay in shape—need not do so.

Some of these stretching exercises may cause—not prevent—injuries. When athletes place a leg up on a bar or a fence and then try to touch their toes, they are straining both the hamstring and the spine. It's almost certain that by doing this regularly, he will eventually develop leg or back problems. This type of warmup doesn't make sense unless it's being performed by a strong, high-level athlete who needs this kind of stretch; it's not recommended for the recreational athlete.

But there is a way to prepare for your run without risking injury. Based on research in the U.S.S.R., this is what I suggest for the recreational jogger: Rather than stretches, run the first mile very slowly. Just take it nice and easy, allowing those muscles to stretch and warm up, and your breathing and body temperature to rise a little at a time. After the first mile, gradually pick up your speed to the pace at which you normally run. This is the best warmup in the world for the kind of running you're doing—and you won't waste time performing unproductive exercises.

The serious athlete, however, *should* go through more formal, traditional warmups. After a ten- to twenty-minute warmup session, he or she can then move into the main exercise period, which is followed by a short (five-minute) cool-down for body restoration.

DYNAMIC ISOMETRICS

Almost everyone has heard of isometric exercises. They became a fad in the 1960s amid claims that startling increases in strength could be achieved with no special equipment,

117

In brief, isometrics involve flexing the muscles against a stationary object — perhaps a wall, or even another muscle. There is no movement at all at the joints. As this flexing occurs, the muscle fibers contract (this isometric contraction is actually 10 percent greater than that which occurs in a concentric contraction). In the process, these fibers attain more strength than before.

Soviet research, however, has learned that the remarkable claims once made for isometrics were overstated. Further, there's a serious problem involved with them: Holding the isometric position for six seconds or more with a maximum contraction places such stress on the muscles, ligaments, and tendons that injuries sometimes occur. Athletes have even blacked out holding their breath too long while performing an isometric contraction.

American coaches proclaimed that isometrics were an extremely effective training method, and by adopting this technique so intensively for a period of time in the 1960s, the Soviets feel their progress was set back about two years. They still use isometrics today, but not nearly to the extent they once did.

Having found flaws in isometric training, the Soviets have created a new system which has already had substantial benefits for the American athletes who have adopted it at my suggestion. This technique can help build strength through the entire range of motion of a joint, as well as work on specific problem areas. Since this new approach involves both movement as well as moments of remaining still, I have coined the name "dynamic isometrics" for it.

In essence, dynamic isometrics combines isometric contractions with eccentric and /or concentric ones. In the weight room, it requires very slow movement using below-maximum levels of weight (60 to 70 percent of maximum), punctuated by brief periods of holding at critical positions. Not only do the weights themselves provide resistance, but gravity plays a role as the weights are lowered.

Here is how to perform a dynamic isometric squat: Begin in the upright position, with the barbell on your shoulders. Then slowly bend the knees, lowering your body until there is about a 160-degree angle in the knee joints (180 degrees is straight, so your knees are barely bent). Hold this position for three to four seconds, and then continue bending slowly at the knees and hips until the knee joints have reached about a 145-degree angle. Hold again for three to four seconds, and then gradually lower yourself once more, stopping and holding for three to four seconds at about a 115-degree angle. Finally, lower yourself again until you reach a 90-degree angle in the knees, and hold again.

After you've held this last position for three to four seconds, you can either rise at a moderate rate of speed, or (if your sport requires explosiveness in the legs) try leaping as high as you can. A maximum of two or three repetitions per training session should be done.

When you perform this dynamic isometric exercise as described here, it takes about twenty to thirty seconds per repetition. Because of the tremendous muscle tension involved, this will seem like an extremely long period of time. But you will really begin to see the benefits after just a few weeks.

Performed in this manner, the squat involves three types of muscular contractions: eccentric (on the way down), isometric (holding in position), and concentric (rising). As I mentioned earlier, you should be placing weights on your shoulders equaling about 60 to 70 percent of the maximum barbell weight you can handle in a single squat. By the time you're done with the exercise, it will feel as though you've been lifting 150 percent of maximum.

Let me add a note of caution: This type of squat can be very taxing. If you experience any tremor while performing it, you have gone beyond what you should be doing. Stop immediately. Make sure you have spotters to help you if problems arise while you're working out.

OTHER SOVIET BREAKTHROUGHS

Here is one Soviet innovation that may be of help to you: as the dynamic isometric squat described above demonstrates, the Soviets have found significant benefit in combining exercises that work on muscles in different ways. There is real value in concentric training, for instance, but to build all-around strength, the muscles should also be worked in eccentric, isometric, and isokinetic ways. In a typical training year, athletes will spend approximately 60 to 70 percent of their time performing concentric exercises (in which the muscles shorten as movement occurs). Another 10 to 15 percent is devoted to eccentric exercises (in which the muscles lengthen), and about the same amount of time is spent on isometrics (in which no change in length takes place). Finally, 5 to 10 percent of the workout schedule is devoted to a variation of isokinetic (or same-speed motion) conditioning,*

As you can see, variety is all important to the Soviets. They have found that it allows for greater gains in strength, probably because it prevents stagnation in the central nervous system which controls the kind of muscular contractions that take place. (The Soviets refer to this as the "nerve-muscle" system.)

According to their research, significant improvements take place when a new exercise is learned because the nervous system is in a state of excitation and responds with a high energy level.

*In the U.S., athletes do their isokinetic exercises only on specialized machines; the Soviets, however, do them with barbells, and thus perform a variation of the isokinetics to which Americans are most accustomed.

Once the body has fully adapted to a particular movement, the nervous system loses this intensity and energy as the exercise is repeated, time after time.

But with a little help from some friends, you can get maximum benefits from exercises by combining two or more of these four methods of gaining strength. Let's assume that your maximum load in performing a squat is 250 pounds. In a standing position, have your assistants put a barbell weighing 300 pounds on your shoulders. Then lower yourself (eccentric) into a squatting position, and remain there for a few moments (isometric). During this stationary period, your two helpers will remove 50 pounds from the bar, bringing the total weight back down to your maximum level. Lastly, you'll return to the standing position (concentric). This kind of exercise takes advantage of the fact that your eccentric strength is 40 to 50 percent greater than your concentric strength, and your isometric strength is 10 to 20 percent superior to your concentric strength.

Earlier in this chapter I mentioned one of several combinations of exercises with which the Soviets have also had a lot of success. It has proven particularly helpful for athletes who need to improve their coordination, from football players to weightlifters. The routine calls for two "good mornings" two squats, and two overhead presses; they vary the number of sets and repetitions, and the speed of execution. Once again, variety is the key.

Combinations of movements are also used in an exercise that has become extremely popular in the U.S.S.R.—the glute-ham-gastroc raise. It is used to strengthen the entire backside —the lower back, buttocks, and hamstrings.

In this exercise, the athlete lies face-down over a gymnastics horse (buck), with the mid-thighs across the horse and the feet secured in nearby wall bars. The head is pointed toward the ground, and the fingers are laced together behind the head (or a barbell is held across the shoulders).

The athlete then raises the trunk up to a straight-body position, using the buttocks and the upper hamstrings. The back is held rigid in that position, or is raised even further into a slight hyperextension. At this point, the athlete flexes the knee joints, allowing the entire body from the knees to be raised even higher, to an angle approximately 45 degrees to the floor. This final movement brings maximal contraction to the hamstrings, and thus is popular with weightlifters, sprinters, and jumpers to help them strengthen and avoid injuries in this region. Unlike typical hamstring contraction exercises, in which only one end of the muscle is in motion, this one involves movement in both ends in sequence.

Unfortunately, the glute-ham-gastroc raise can be difficult to perform without special equipment. Several years ago, I invented an apparatus for use with this particular exercise. Called the Glute-Ham Developer, it is now available in the U.S. in many sporting goods stores and from Sports Training, Inc.

Note, however, that variety in a conditioning program does not always require the complex merger of exercises or movements. In fact, you can perform exactly the same maneuver first on free weights and then on a machine, to achieve some subtle but important changes in the way the nervous system responds. Changes in the number of sets or repetitions, or in the resistance, can make a difference, too, giving the central nervous system time to regenerate and prepare for new, higher performance levels. Some research shows that, as a general rule, you should incorporate some changes into your exercise schedule every three to four weeks.

Along with such innovations in sports training, the Soviets also continue making a special effort to prevent and minimize the seriousness of sports injuries. Lower back pain is as prevalent in the U.S.S.R. as in the West, and most Soviet data show that changes in the intervertebral disks are usually the cause of this pain among athletes, which often begins after jumping to the ground from a height. While walking, the spine experiences a force of one-half to one unit of gravity with each step, but when a gymnast jumps from a horizontal bar onto a thin layer of mats, the force can be as much as 10 *g.*

To reduce the incidence of back injuries among their athletes, the Soviets now encourage them to work on strengthening the muscles of the lumbar region — in essence, to create a muscular corset around their midsection that will help with-stand the forces received by this area of the spine. To develop these abdominal muscles, many of their athletes now routinely perform leg raises with the torso securely anchored or while hanging from an overhead bar, (For individuals whose backs are already weak, sit-ups with the legs bent are the best choice.)

The back muscles can be strengthened with exercises such as the spinal extension, in which the upper body hangs over the end of a table, and is then raised to a slightly arched position. For the deep muscles of the back, stand with your back to the wall so that the heels, buttocks, shoulders, and head touch it. Then, while keeping these parts against the wall, try straightening the spine so the lumbar region presses against the wall and even exerts pressure on it. During each workout session, perform five to six repetitions of this exercise, each lasting four to five seconds. If it's too difficult at first, try it while lying on the floor on your back; once you've mastered it there, return to the standing position.

I rely on Soviet techniques like these when I work with athletes in the U.S. Here is another example. Several years ago I began working with Todd Marinovich, then a freshman high school quarterback who was throwing the football about forty yards. I was convinced that his arm could be made stronger and more powerful. A close analysis of the passing motion— using Soviet descriptions of throwing actions for maximum distance—provided the key to strengthening his throwing arm,

Here's how we did it: Weight training is not uncommon for quarterbacks in the U.S., but they often do it in unproductive ways that provide little if any extra strength for their passing attack. They frequently begin pulley exercises, for example, with the upper arm in line with the shoulder, and the lower arm at a right angle to the ground, pointing toward the ceiling. Then they will tug the apparatus forward, imitating the passing motion.

However, the power required for passing is actually needed earlier in the motion, beginning at the point where the arm is cocked all the way back, almost parallel to the ground. So by starting the exercise when the arm is perpendicular to the ground, which most Americans do, they are concentrating almost exclusively on the follow-through, not the actual throwing itself. Analysis makes it clear that medial-shoulder-joint-rotation work is what is really needed.

So I had Todd use a barbell, and begin the exercise with his arm cocked all the way back. This was a much closer simulation of his actual passing motion. Before long, his throwing strength started to improve.

Todd was also introduced to explosive training for legs, arms, and total body. He used various forms of these "plyometric" exercises (see Chapter Five), including throwing and catching a series of medicine balls in various ways, providing variable resistance for maximum speed. I also noticed that the leg exercises that had been prescribed for him were threatening to cause some serious back damage, so I recommended that he eliminate them and substitute simple squats instead,

Todd also added some midsection rotation or twisting exercises to his program, like the Russian twist. He began doing leg abductions, too, to help him step into the throw, as well as to help him make quick movements to the side if needed for escaping the rush. He's now throwing passes that sometimes measure over seventy yards, and I believe that the best may be yet to come.

Chapter 4 Addendum

Before moving on to additional innovations that have been uncovered since the original book was published, it is important that you first read or re-read the original chapter. It presents excellent background for the updated information that will now be discussed in the same order as it appears in the basic text.

Periodization

The concept of periodization is still basically the same although much has changed in the actual periodization schemes. This has been precipitated by the increased amount of competition in which most professional—and to a good extent scholastic—athletes are now engaged. Because of the greater amount of competition there is less time to train. Thus, the training time must be precise and productive and there can be little if any wasted time. This is especially true for the high level athlete who is literally forced to modify and change his periodization scheme to get more work done in less time. In addition his training time must be even more productive than in the typical annual or semi-annual periodization scheme.

One factor in periodization that stands out among all others, is the need for greater individualization. According to many of the top Russian researchers and coaches, there are now many different periodization schemes based mainly on the type of athlete, how he responds to training and his sport. They have identified well over 150 schematics, the use of which depends on the athlete and how he responds to the different types of trainings. However, the basic tenets of periodization still remain the same. Each athlete must go through four stages (GPP, SPP, competition, transition) regardless of how long each stage may last. Thus the key variable in the contemporary periodization scheme is the amount of time spent in each phase and the exact kind of training done. Note that it is quite different for elite and novice athletes as well as older and younger athletes.

The Russian's often call each phase of the general (GPP) and specialized (SPP) training period, the phase of sports form development. This means that regardless of whether the high level athlete is doing GPP or SPP, at the end of each specific phase he should reach a top level of sports form, i.e., he should peak in the development of whatever qualities and/or skills he is working on during this particular phase. When the athlete goes through a GPP phase that lasts anywhere from two to six weeks, he should "max-out" in regard to his development. The SPP phase can also last the same or greater amount of time and can lead into another specialized phase that blends into the pre-competitive or competitive period. In essence, each phase can have two or more stages depending on the level of the athlete.

If the high level athlete is looking for additional development in only one or two physical qualities it would require use of a block program in the specialized physical preparation phase. The block concept is probably the latest innovation which has proven to be very successful in achieving greater development of any one or two physical qualities that the athlete needs. Usually it is greater specific strength, speed-strength or speed that the power athlete is trying to achieve or muscular aerobic and/or anaerobic endurance for the endurance athlete.

Since the original book came out, there has been discussion in regard to whether the periodization plan should show straight line improvement or if the improvement should be wave like in nature. For the most part, these concepts are immaterial as they depend on how the athlete reacts to the different types of training and in which phase he is working. Thus, progress made by each individual athlete can take on one or another (or both) forms. They may show combinational progress, one phase may be straight line, then it may level off and could be wave like in another. In all cases, however, when progress is mapped out over the year, you should see constant progress. This is the key element that should be looked at. For additional information on periodization, see articles in the Soviet Sports Review, especially those by Dr. Anatoly Bondarchuk.

General Preparatory Period (GPP)

The explanation of general physical preparation as outlined in the original book still holds true today. However, it applies more to the novice but bonafide athlete. The reason for this is that the today's high level athlete maintains his fitness throughout the year so that he does not have to go through an extensive preparatory period to "get in shape". [Note that with this definition, most professional baseball and to a great extent, football players would not qualify as elite or high level]. As a result, the GPP for the high level athlete is shorter, more concentrated and usually focused more on physical qualities that are lagging or in need of rehabilitation.

A distinction must be made here between general preparatory exercises and general developmental exercises. The developmental exercises are used to improve specific physical qualities and/or skills and are not geared to all-round physical preparation. In GPP you strengthen the overall body which may or may not show improved sports performance which is usually reserved for the SPP phase. The main thrust of GPP is to prepare the body for the more intense training that occurs in the specialized period or before doing developmental exercises.

It should also be noted that GPP for novice athletes should include concentrated technique training. It is at this time that skills should be improved. Technique work is also done by the high level athlete even though his skills are fairly well formed. Because of increases in strength and other physical qualities, there will be changes in technique. As a result, more technique work is done in the specialized period so that the gains made in strength and other physical qualities will be incorporated into the skill execution, to make it even more effective. Thus for the higher level athlete, technique improvement comes in the SPP phase while for novice athletes it falls mainly in GPP and continues through SPP.

According to the Russians, one should never separate technique from development of physical abilities. The two should always go hand in hand. Sadly in the U.S., technique is too often ignored while physical training, especially strength training, is overemphasized. There are many reasons for this but most prevalent is that most coaches do not understand skill technique. They are not to be faulted for this because it is not taught and they never have an opportunity to learn about technique when they played.

The myth that coaches should not "fix it if it ain't broke" should be busted. Everyone can improve their technique, even at the highest world class levels. I learned this soon after I started reading the Soviet track and field journal track for coaches. In every issue they had a cinematogram of a world-class runner, jumper or thrower. They also had a frame by frame analysis of the athlete's technique. Because of my background in biomechanics I was very interested in these analyses. However when comparing the text to the respective photos in the cinematogram, I did not always see what they were talking about. To me the technique looked good. After all these were world-class athletes, many of whom had world records.

However, after about a year of reading and rereading these articles, the light finally came on and I began to understand the analyses and to see exactly what they were discussing. They brought out very fine points of the technique and even made recommendations on how they could be improved or corrected with special exercises. These readings gave me a much better understanding of what is involved on the highest levels of technique execution. It has enabled me to pick out even the smallest errors in technique that would ordinarily be missed.

For example, the top female marathoner in the U.S. at the present time is Deena Kastor who still has a major flaw in her running technique. She is a heel hitter which is very inefficient and possibly injury producing. In addition, she does not have sufficient muscular endurance of the hip flexors to maintain the same stride throughout the race. But yet no one has corrected or taught her to run more efficiently and effectively. Until then, I hope that she does not experience any problems. More importantly however, is that with a correction in her technique she could be faster, experience less fatigue and as a result, be even more dominant in the running world.

As I became more proficient in looking at all levels of athletes and especially runners, I put this information together in a book called Explosive Running. Not only does it contain biomechanical analyses of different level runnerrs supported by sequence pictures taken from live digital film, but a chapter devoted to common running errors and how they can be corrected with specialized and/or explosive exercises. The book is easy to read but as with me, it may take a second or third reading of selected sections to fully comprehend all of the information presented.

Specialized Physical Preparation (SPP)

The general concept of SPP and the exercises described in the original book hold true to this day. One factor that was omitted, however, was that most of the exercises should duplicate what occurs in execution in part or a good portion of the sports skill. The descriptions for some of the exercises were based on developing the physical abilities, specific to the sports event. However, to make the exercises even more specialized, they should be modified to duplicate the motor pathway and muscle contraction regime.

This is a very important concept that should not be ignored. According to the Russians, when an exercise duplicates a portion of the total skill or a single joint action, the athlete will gain strength, speed-strength (or other physical quality) as it is displayed in execution of the competitive sports skill. In this way, both technique and the physical abilities are developed simultaneously and impact performance in a positive way. The improvement is much greater than if only one factor were trained.

When you do an exercise, as for example, for greater strength in the same range of motion and in the same neuromuscular pathway as used in execution of a skill, then you also develop a muscular feel for the action in addition to increasing strength. This enables you to recognize effective performance and makes it possible to repeat the skill in competition. Such exercises show almost immediate improvement!

This concept can be better illustrated with a running specific exercise called the knee or thigh drive. This exercise is specific to running, because when the thigh is brought forward the hip flexor muscle action begins when the thigh is at its furthestmost point to the rear. The leg reaches this point behind the body after the push-off when it is moving backward in relation to the upper body. The hip flexor muscle activity continues to pull the thigh forward until the thigh is directly below the body, in a vertical position. The muscle activity then diminishes and the hamstrings come into play (eccentrically) to eventually stop the forward thigh movement after it reaches its furthest forward-upward point. The exact height that the thigh achieves is determined by how forcefully the thigh is accelerated forward.

This leg action is duplicated in an exercise with Active Cords. An ankle strap is placed around the ankle and 1-3 Active cords, the exact tension depending on the strength of the athlete--are then attached thigh high to a stationary beam or post. The athlete then assumes a position in which the thigh is as far behind the body as possible and there is strong tension in the cords with the knee bent and the shin level. As the athlete feels strong tension on the hip flexors he then drives the knee forward to a position of about 30-40 degrees in front of the body. It is not necessary to drive the knee upward as this is an unwanted and un-needed action.

This exercise duplicates what occurs in the running stride. It develops the muscles over the range of motion in which they are active in the running stride. As a result, doing this exercise and other running specific exercises, show almost an immediate positive effect on running performance. Athletes who have done this exercise have found definite increases in their running speed and depending upon the number of repetitions and the tension used, improvement in maintaining speed over the distance.

For example, many runners use this exercise to develop muscular endurance so that they can maintain good form and running speed throughout the entire race, especially in the 400, 800 and greater distance races. In my research I have found that most runners who begin to slow down in the latter part of their race do so because of their inability to drive the thigh forward with the same intensity and range of motion as they do when they first begin the race. Thus, this exercise helps to ensure that they're able to maintain good running technique – and speed--through the entire race. This is another example of how understanding effective technique—and applying the knowledge—can make better coaches and athletes.

Many more exercises can be described here but I hope this is sufficient to show the concept of a true specialized exercise. For more information on running specific exercises, see *Explosive Running.* For more information on technique and specialized exercises for other basic sports skills, it is recommended that you read *Build a Better Athlete, Explosive Basketball Training, Explosive Golf, Explosive Tennis,* and *Women's Soccer: Using Science to Improve Speed.*

To get the most out of your specialized physical preparation be sure that most of the exercises duplicate what occurs in execution of your sports skill. The major criteria, somewhat modified from the original text, that you should keep in mind are as follows:

1. The exercise must duplicate the neuromuscular pathway seen in execution of the competitive skill.
2. Strength must be developed in the same range of motion as it is displayed in the execution of the competitive skill.
3. The exercise must involve the same type of muscular contraction as used in execution of the competitive skill.

These are the main criteria that most coaches can use although there are still others that can be applied. When you do such specialized exercises you experience the true meaning of conjugate training. This means that strength is developed as it is used in the skill technique execution, i.e., technique is coupled with strength in its display. Conjugate also means the coupling of two different type exercises as for example, a strength exercise followed by an explosive strength exercise. But even in this context it is necessary that the exercises duplicate the same action seen in execution of the sports skill. It is not simply the coupling of any two exercises; they must overlap in their effect.

For example, a maximum effort strength exercise should activate the nervous system in exactly the same way that it will be involved in the explosive exercise. In essence you are doing the same thing (using the same neuro-muscular pathway) but you rely on the nervous system imprint from the strength exercise to execute the explosive exercise. In this way, you can get an even stronger contraction of the muscles in the explosive exercise. However, keep mind that this type of exercise is highly stressful. It should not be used by novices; it is intended only for high level athletes and only in SPP, in the pre-competitive period.

Competitive Period

The competitive period involves mostly competition and preparation for competition. Thus, considerable time is spent on strategy and tactics and preparing for the opponent. According to the Russians it should not be a period for greater increases in strength or other physical qualities except in some individual sports where this is required as for example, in the iron sports and to limited extent in some track and field events.

However, the concept of in-season increases in strength is still quite prevalent in the U.S. But maintenance of strength should be more important especially in the team sports. In this case, the athlete still does strength exercises, but not for greater amounts of strength, training is aimed at maintaining the achieved levels of the various physical qualities needed. The reason for this is that if there are any strength gains or losses in-season, it will interfere with technique execution. Exhibiting good technique should be paramount in any training during the competitive period. You must maintain the strength levels that you achieved in order to most effectively execute the game skills and as a result, better carry out the strategy and as a result, excel in the competition.

Also important in the competitive period is recovery and restoration. All too often athletes do not have sufficient rest or do not use recovery methods to get over the exertion or physical abuse that their bodies may undergo during competition and more often in training. This is especially true in sports such as American football. This is why it is surprising that more teams do not make greater use of restorative measures. Most often only whirlpools are used but mainly for injury treatment, not for recovery. There are many other water type treatments that can be successfully used as for example, Jacuzzis, different types of showers, (Sharko) underwater massage, etc. that are excellent for recovery. For more information on the many restoration measures available see chapter 9 in this book and *Sports Restoration and Massage*.

Transitional (Post Competition) Period

Very little can be added to what is already described in the original book. Suffice it to say that this period is extremely important for all athletes and especially high level athletes. According to the Russians, regardless of how long a cycle of sports form development may last, the athlete should <u>always</u> have a period of restoration in between. A one week or more transitional period is a must, especially after the last major competition or competitive period. If there is no competition, the transitional period can be much less but again it will depend upon the type and length of training and competition. Also, in general, the older the athlete, the longer the recovery period.

Periodization in the U.S.?

Periodization is already widely accepted in the U.S. Most teams and strength coaches employ some form of periodization in the training of their athletes. In general, these periodization plans follow the basic format outlined in the original text or its' variants. As more information becomes available, some coaches are beginning to modify their periodization concepts and training plans. As brought out earlier, the exact changes in the periodization schemes depend on the athlete, his sport, level of mastery etc.

It is also necessary to re-emphasize the need for a multi-year periodization scheme for up-and-coming athletes. This periodization scheme begins in the early years, known as the period of universal preparation. This means that the youngster is exposed to a wide variety of sports and other activities to develop all the basic physical abilities, coordinations, movement patterns, sports skills, etc. The development of this base takes five to six years during which the youngster is still involved in playing sports, but not specializing in any.

The key point, according to the Russians, is that the youngsters should be involved in a variety of activities to develop the foundation which will then allow them to become the best possible in any one sport as an adult. Sadly, the trend in the U.S. is in the opposite direction. We see more and more early specialization and more youngsters dropping out of the sport when teenagers.

They do not continue playing to become the best possible when adults. Part of this is due to the boredom of only playing one sport and part is due to their inability to improve significantly after passing puberty and significant maturation.

The concept of early specialization probably originated from the erroneous reporting in the media stating that the former Soviets and East Germans literally took the youngster out of the crib to make him an athlete. This could not be further from the truth. But it was sensationalized and had a major impact on coaches and parents. It is possible to see a distinct change in player development when this myth became firmly established. The main focus was and still remains on more playing and competing in the early years—not on training.

The Russians believe that specialization in most sports should not begin until the ages of 12-14. Earlier participation should be mainly to learn technique, and to develop physical abilities, coordination, etc. Once technique is mastered in the exercises and in the skills that the youngster will need, they will then be ready to get involved in more high intensity training. The results at this time will be both rapid and very dramatic. But if specialization is started at an early age, progress will be slow mainly because it takes longer to develop the coordination and other physical qualities that are needed to master and perfect not only older, but new skills.

The Russians found that complete athletic mastery and high level performance should take place when the athlete is in his late teenage years or early 20's, older in some sports. Earlier specialization usually leads to failure; only in rare cases is it successful. Exceptions to this can be found in sports such as figure skating and gymnastics.

Flexibility

Because little has changed in the area of flexibility since the first book came out, I would like to reemphasize some of the more important points brought out. First is that active stretching is much more effective than static stretching. If static stretching is done over a prolonged period of time, it can be detrimental and may even be the culprit in causing many injuries. Second is that static stretches, in which you hold the end position for up to 60 or more seconds, are great for increasing your range of motion but if this extra range of motion is not needed, it will not enhance your performance. Instead it has a great possibility of decreasing your ability active to perform well because of overstretched ligaments and resultant weaker joints.

Third, active stretches for sport should be very specific to the joint actions that occur in execution of the skills. In other words, the exercises should duplicate the movements seen in each of the major joint actions. They should mimic what the athletes does in the sports.

For example, doing the good morning exercise is very effective for both stretching and strengthening the hamstring muscle, which is important for runners and athletes who run in their sport as in soccer, baseball, football, etc. Doing a forward lunge in the classical manner (also known as the Russian lunge) in which you take a very long stride and maintain an erect upper body position, is very effective for stretching the hip joint flexors that play the key role in driving the thigh forward for running speed.

Many more exercises can be described here, but suffice it to say that most of them are already in the literature. For example, if you're interested in more running specific stretches, see *Explosive Running*. If your sport is basketball, see the specific active stretches for basketball in *Explosive Basketball Training*. At least one chapter is devoted to specific stretches for that particular sport in the other sports training books by Dr. Yessis.

Recent research is proving that tighter muscles may be safer than looser muscles and joints. For example, studies have shown that professional basketball players have tighter hamstrings which appears to be needed for better performances. This is understandable since when they are tighter, they are ready to be more quickly involved in running, cutting, jumping, etc. If they are loose, they cannot tense sufficiently in the shortest time to exhibit explosive power. As is well known, quickness comes from prior tensing of the muscles and quick reversals—from eccentric to concentric. The looser the joint or muscle is, the longer it takes to produce maximum force. Tighter muscles can react more quickly.

This finding substantiates the need for active stretching to activate the muscles and get them ready to perform as well as to increase the range of motion in healthy athletes. The key element here is that flexibility must be accompanied with strength when increasing range of motion. This allows the muscle to function more effectively and to react quicker and more powerfully when executing various game skills.

Dynamic Isometrics

Dynamic isometrics is now known as explosive isometrics. The example using the squat exercise for dynamic isometrics has been somewhat modified over the years but doing the exercises as described is still valid and beneficial. However, because of the great tension that is built up in the muscles, such exercises are recommended only at the end of a workout. If done early in the workout, the muscles will become too fatigued to allow you to have a quality workout with other exercises or activities.

In explosive isometrics you assume a position where the muscle is placed on stretch as in the beginning of a power (explosive) movement and you then hold this position as tension builds up for up to four to five seconds. When the tension is sufficiently strong, quickly explode and move the limb or body as quickly as possible.

For example, if doing the knee drive exercise, have someone hold the leg behind you (or use high tension Active Cords) while you hold an upright position. The person holding your foot should be pulling backwards while you resist it by pulling forward, creating great tension in the hip flexors. After 4-5 seconds the person holding the leg back releases it and you automatically drive forward with maximum speed. The key element here is to get a powerful initial contraction at the beginning of the range of motion. This is needed to quickly accelerate the limb to develop maximum speed of movement.

This exercise can also be done with Active Cords in which you create sufficient tension on the muscles with the cords by standing far enough away from the stationary attachment or using multiple cords with the leg behind you. Once you have great tension while you remain in an erect standing position, resist for up to 4-5 seconds and then quickly drive the thigh forward. In this case, because of the great tension, you may not be able to drive the thigh very far forward. This is not a problem, since your main objective is to initiate acceleration, not to maintain speed through the full motion.

Other examples of doing explosive isometrics can be found in the bench press where you hold the down position for 4-5 seconds with a fairly heavy bar and then quickly try to accelerate the bar upward. Since many sporting moves involve elbow extension, begin with the elbow in a bent position, about halfway through the range of motion. Then quickly initiate an explosive movement upward. If needed, the bar can be released but then you must be able to catch it as it descends and then hold it on extended arms after absorbing the initial shock of receiving the barbell.

Other Soviet Breakthroughs

Most of the Soviet breakthroughs have already been mentioned. Since the former Soviet Union was broken up soon after the printing of the original book, there haven't been any additional major innovations. However, in regard to some of the concepts mentioned, a few additional words are warranted in regard to the central nervous system (CNS).

The Russians have found that stress to the nervous system may be more important than stress to the muscles or body. The reason for this is that the nervous system controls the actions performed by the athlete. It must be in a high state of energy in order for the athlete to perform well. If the nervous system is sluggish, the athlete will not perform well. Thus, recovery and recuperation are very important for the nervous system.

Exercises such as depth jumps are especially hard on the CNS. Russian studies have shown that even though depth jumps appear to be relatively easy, their affect on the CNS is extremely great. Athletes often experience poor sleep, poor appetites, and general discomfort. It can take up to two days to fully recover. This is why deviating from the prescribed protocol such as going over thirty inches in height, or doing too many sets, can prove to be potentially disruptive.

Training should revolve around CNS energy. When you first begin a workout, your nervous system is typically fresh and ready to perform. Thus, the beginning of the workout becomes the best time to do technique and/or speed work, after an appropriate warmup. In essence, all technique work should be done only when the nervous system is fully energized. Strength training can be done when in a fatigue state but it should not be excessive fatigue. Endurance training can be done at the end of a workout when there is fatigue. Thus, select the type of training that you do around the ability of the nervous system to perform at its best, which then allows the body to perform at its best.

In regard to the Glute-Ham Developer (GHD) that I created and the glute-ham gastroc raise exercise(g-h-g) exercise I got from the Russians, there are now many companies making this machine for this exercise. However, many of them, because of their poor understanding of how this and other exercises should be executed, make inadequate machines. There are too many glute-ham machines that are potentially harmful to the athlete mainly because they do not allow for proper positioning or have adjustments that are too difficult to make (or cannot be made). But correct positioning is critical for effective execution of not only the glute-ham gastroc raise but the abdominal and lower back exercises. Because of what should be strict manufacturing guidelines, I have found it difficult to find a manufacturer that will make an effective one.

For information on how the g-h-g raise and other exercises should be done, see *Kinesiology of Exercise*. Note that these exercises are extremely important for athletes. For example, the back raise which is best done on the GHD, is probably the best lower back exercise available for strengthening the lumbar muscles through their full range of motion. Note that a Roman Chair and some Glute Hams are not adjustable and fit only people of average or short heights. Thus, for tall persons, doing the back raise can be injurious on some machines. In addition, two variants of the full range abdominal exercises are best done on a GHD to duplicate the muscle action seen in running and for other actions seen in volleyball (spike), basketball (fall away jump shot) and soccer (throw in).

A few additional comments should also be made in regard to Todd Marinovich, the young quarterback that I trained. I began with him when he was 13 years old and directed his training up until he quit the university and signed a professional contract with the LA Raiders. Soon after the printing of the book, Todd broke most high school records for passing. But, it appears that he was unable to handle the freedom that he was exposed to while at USC. He got involved in the drug scene and even to this day is having problems with drugs. It is a sad commentary for a fine athlete who could have achieved extraordinary greatness had he continued his training and followed a better pathway. The training technique analysis and the exercises that I prescribed for him were quite unique at that time and can serve any quarterback well even to this day. For information on training the quarterback see the DVD, *Specialized Strength and Explosive Exercises for the Quarterback.*

Chapter 5:

SPEED-STRENGTH TRAINING: A New Soviet Breakthrough

If you're a high jumper or a basketball player, would you like to be able to add an extra 3 to 6 inches to the height you're presently able to leap? Or if you're a swimmer, would you like to slice a few seconds off your time in the 200-meter freestyle? If you run 10-kilometer races, would you savor cutting a minute off your best time to date? Or if you play football or tennis, would you like to make quicker movements and cutting actions?

These are the kinds of goals that can be accomplished with speed-strength (explosive) training, probably the most significant innovation developed by Soviet sports researchers in recent years. This technique is gradually being introduced in the U.S., where it's most commonly known as "plyometrics." I consider it the wave of the future.

In short, speed-strength exercises are designed to develop explosiveness in athletes so they can execute movements as rapidly as possible, while still also exhibiting strength. These are characteristics important in a wide range of sports, from running and racquetball to baseball and weightlifting.

In baseball or football, for instance, the goal of the pitcher or the quarterback is to accelerate his arm so rapidly that the ball zips forward at maximum speed or distance. The shot-putter is aiming for the same thing—that is, to ensure that the 16-pound shot is moving at maximum speed when it is released. Gymnasts need both arm and leg explosiveness, and the baseball batter requires rapid movements of the arms and trunk.

Although speed-strength is important in most sports, the training itself is almost always conducted in the weight room or on a throwing field. It was once rare to find anyone but weightlifters pumping iron, but now nearly everyone does it, no matter what the sport. In the U.S., however, weights have been used almost exclusively to develop strength alone, not explosiveness.

Of course, neither I nor the Soviets would argue against the value of enhancing strength. But research in the U.S.S.R. has concluded that there's more to success in sports than strength. Javelin throwers, for instance, must move their hands forward with maximum speed and acceleration. The volleyball player at the net must leap with both speed and explosiveness.

People should think of their muscles as rubber bands. When explosiveness has been developed, there is first a forced stretching and tensing of the muscles, after which the energy from this "loading" switches directions (as though the rubber band were snapping back), unloading the muscles as it propels the body upward or forward.

Ideally, a sprinter's foot is in contact with the ground for only one-tenth of a second; a high jumper using the "Fosbury flop" technique keeps his foot on the ground for just two-tenths of a second before takeoff. Thus, the muscles must release with maximal force in an instant.

Recent Soviet studies show that while strength is an important foundation for avoiding injuries, it is beneficial only up to a point for enhancing explosiveness. If you're doing strength training for the first time, your enhanced strength will undoubtedly make you a better athlete. But over the years, if you concentrate only on strength, this can eventually become a detriment, not an aid, to performance.

Powerlifting, for example, involves slow strength movements. The weight is at maximum levels, and with the exercises being performed in a deliberate fashion, athletes can achieve impressive gains in strength and muscle mass. But there's a catch: while they're gaining strength, they simultaneously lose speed. In essence, their nervous system and body learn slowness. Thus, there must be a cutoff point, after which the athlete moves from strength into explosiveness training.

In the U.S., however, strength training is just about the only game in town. We still tend to believe that maximum strength is synonymous with superior performance—the stronger you are, the better athlete you'll be.

But you can frequently see the actual outcome of these beliefs on the playing field. In football, for example, linemen have trained with heavier and heavier weights, and brag that they can bench-press 500 or 600 pounds. However, show me an athlete who can bench-press 600 pounds, and I'll show you someone moving like a tortoise. A football lineman does need strength, but too many overdo it. In their quest for larger muscles, they become heavier, bulkier—and slower.

But maximum weight levels do more than just slow athletes down. Recent Soviet studies show that they may also become more injury-prone. As I've suggested earlier, the athlete who works out places a continuous and severe strain upon the ligaments, tendons, and other muscle support tissues. These tissues simply may not be able to handle such extreme levels of weight. Over time, they weaken, and as they do, the risk of injury escalates.

What is the alternative? Rather than seeking to build only muscle, why not go for some explosiveness as well? In general, strength is developed by using high resistance and low repetitions. By contrast, though, speed and explosiveness require a different tactic—relatively low resistance and rapid execution.

In combining both strength and speed training, the key is to concentrate initially on strength building and then, after a period of weeks or months, to switch to lower weights and faster movements. You need to form a base of strength, but once it has been developed and the first signs of slowing down appear, you should then begin working on speed, and only maintain your strength at its existing level. With the lighter weights, the movement patterns are often identical to those used in strength training, but the exercises are done much more rapidly, with more repetitions, and with adequate rest in between. (A few athletes can continue to increase their strength without any decline in speed; for them, a strength-training program can continue in earnest.)

I've now read dozens of studies on speed-strength training conducted in the U.S.S.R., and I'm sold on it. There's no doubt in my mind that it is effective. One paper after another has shown that this unique approach to training dramatically improves the athlete's reactiveness and explosiveness.

Why is speed-strength training so effective? Yuri Verhoshansky is the leading Soviet researcher into speed-strength (our plyometrics). His research has shown that, to a large degree, these exercises work on the so-called fast-twitch muscle fibers, which the athlete relies upon for quick movements while competing. In effect, speed training recruits these muscle fibers from within the body, and provokes maximum stimulation and frequency of firing. (These fast-twitch fibers draw their name from their ability to produce a maximum muscle contraction much faster than slow-twitch fibers can, thus explaining their capacity for explosiveness.)

Therefore, on top of the strength that has been built up, the athlete can now add the important element of enhanced muscle reactiveness. The switch from strength to speed training also brings some variety into an athlete's training program, which has both physical and psychological benefits. While preventing boredom and mental fatigue from setting in, it also keeps the body from becoming overly comfortable. As coaches may have told you, if you do only one type of workout, month after month, improvement virtually ceases.

Speed-strength training dates back only to the 1960s. It had its beginnings with Soviet track-and-field athletes, particularly the jumpers, who found that their performances became much better with increases in explosiveness. Then athletes and coaches in other sports gradually began taking notice of it, and today its benefits can be seen in the performances of athletes in nearly every sport in the Eastern-bloc countries. Research carried out on one area — track and field — has been applied to many others, a phenomenon almost unheard of in the U.S.

CREATING A SPEED-STRENGTH PROGRAM

If you seem to lack the explosiveness that your sport calls for, you should consider incorporating plyometric training into your own workouts. As far as can be determined, explosive power must be developed through speed-strength training; although some people are born with it, even they must still train to elicit their full abilities. Here are some guidelines to get you going, regardless of your innate talent.

The Strength Component

When training for strength *and* speed, both elements are occasionally developed simultaneously. But in most instances, they are worked on in sequence, starting with strength.

I believe that regardless of your sport or level of fitness, you should be developing strength first. There's a good reason for this. When the shift is ultimately made to explosiveness training, the forces created in these exercises reach as much as twenty times your body weight. To withstand such forces, you must already have concentric, eccentric, and isometric strength.

In general, this strength-building period should take one to three months and be performed once or twice a year, depending upon whether you enter major competitions. Once a minimum strength base has been established, speed training can begin.

Although no specific strength program applies to everyone, you should think in terms of all-around conditioning, using many different exercises that incorporate many different movements. For some suggestions on specific exercises that would be appropriate here, refer back to Chapter Four for a list of exercises helpful for general preparatory training. In the weight room, concentrate on training with near-maximum weight (that is, 75 to 90 percent of the most you can lift in one repetition of a particular exercise).

Because the weight is so great, the exercises themselves have to be performed slowly, with only a few repetitions at a time. Generally, several sets of each exercise should be scheduled for a single training session; these will completely exhaust the muscles and bring about the greatest increases in muscle mass and strength.

As a guideline, two to four near-maximum repetitions will develop only strength (without muscle mass). By raising the number of repetitions to five to ten, you'll get both strength and mass. By increasing to ten to twenty repetitions, muscle mass will receive the primary attention, with less emphasis upon strength. And over twenty repetitions will move you much more into muscular endurance rather than muscle mass.

Once your general strength base is well developed, then you can concentrate on strength exercises that closely duplicate the actual movements involved in your sport. The more specific the exercises, the greater the effectiveness of your workout.

Here are some guidelines to follow in creating this part of your exercise program:

1. The exercises should correspond—by form and muscle work—to the action involved in your sport. The range of motion must be the same as in the sport.

2. The strength exercises must correspond to the direction of movement in your sport. For instance, in sprinting, the pushoff leg moves toward the rear; thus, the exercise movement should be directed toward the rear as well.

3. Select exercises where the maximum effort occurs at the same point in the range of motion as in your sport. If you're a runner, your maximum effort takes place when you begin to bring the thigh of your swing leg forward with hip-joint flexion; the force diminishes after the leg passes underneath the body. Thus, when working out, select exercises where your maximum effort occurs at the beginning of the movement, letting inertia carry the limb the rest of the way.

The Speed Component

After up to three months of strength training, it's time to switch gears. Essentially, you'll be moving to lighter weights (30 to 50 percent of maximum). And as the loads decrease, the speed of execution increases. The emphasis here should be on quick (explosive) movements.

During this period, the strength you've already achieved will not be lost. Furthermore, your body will recuperate faster from your exercise sessions, making this a sensible training regimen to continue with right up to—and even during—the competitive season itself.

As you work on developing maximum muscular explosion, you have to be psyched prior to the explosive moment. The exercise requires maximum effort; in fact, the effort should be greater than what is needed during actual performance or competition itself. By approaching the exercise this way, the nervous system will experience the speed being generated, and then will find it easier to approach or duplicate this speed in competition.

Several of the exercises described in Chapter Four can be utilized during speed training. Some will help you develop leg explosiveness; others are for arm explosiveness; still others can work on the total body. In all cases, however, they should be performed with less weight and more rapidity.

Also, I suggest that you incorporate some additional exercises that the Soviets have found particularly helpful in speed training — namely, various jumps, such as single and double leg hopping, depth jumps, and leg push-offs, as well as arm push-offs, arm depth jumps, and catching and throwing medicine balls to work on upper body (and arm) explosiveness. These specific exercises prepare your muscles for the fastest contractions — the kind of activity that you need in competition in most sports. This is high-intensity training, in which powerful muscular contractions are called for in response to the stretching (or dynamic loading) of the involved muscles.

Then it's time to try some depth jumps. But before performing the kind described below, be sure you have already developed sufficient strength in your ankles, knees, hips, back, shoulders, and arms. Weakness in these joints could result in injury. In effect, these exercises will force you to handle abnormally high resistance, equivalent to several times your body weight.

Here is how to execute one of the most effective types of depth jumps, utilizing what is called the "hit" or "shock" method: stand on a bench or a box approximately 30 to 40 inches (but only 12 to 20 inches if you're just beginning) off the ground. Then, with your back held straight, take a long step outward and drop vertically to the floor, with your feet about hip-width apart. The landing should be vertical to create maximum loading on the muscles.

As soon as you hit the ground, the leg extensor muscles will automatically contract eccentrically to resist the downward force. The instant your downward motion stops (but not before), you should then jump as high as possible. The key here is a rapid upward jump, changing the contraction from eccentric to concentric. The faster you switch from loading to take-off, the greater the height, the explosiveness — and the benefit.

Be certain that you have chosen a relatively soft or resilient surface to land on, such as a weightlifting mat or a gymnastics or wrestling mat. Also, in the landing, the balls of the feet should touch the ground first, followed by the whole foot. Only then should there be ankle, knee, and hip-joint flexion.

You can also better prepare yourself for the high leap upward by concentrating on it prior to your jump, thinking "leap up" before hitting the ground. In other words, prepare yourself for the landing and takeoff before they happen. Get yourself "psyched up" to make the fastest and most forceful jump possible.

These jumps are usually performed in a series of ten, three times a week, with the height gradually increasing over time. The ideal height is in the 30-to-40-inch range. At the 30-inch plateau, most of the emphasis is on speed; from 40 inches, there's some shift to strength as well. In any event, always start at a low level—from 12 to 20 inches—and gradually work your way up.

The key to explosive training lies in the stretching and tensing of the muscle prior to its contraction. The faster the stretch or the greater the amount of muscle tension, the greater the explosive power displayed. In the depth jump, for example, here is the sequence of events that takes place.

Immediately upon landing, the extensor muscles of the ankle, knee, and hip joints undergo contraction to stop the body from collapsing onto the floor. In so doing, they undergo slight flexion, which is controlled by the eccentric contraction of the extensor muscles. During this contraction, the extensor muscles lengthen—that is, while the muscle fibers are striving to shorten, the force of the landing is so great it actually lengthens the muscle as it undergoes contraction.

The Soviets have their own way of describing this action. They say the muscle yields to the force—that is, the eccentric contraction is a yielding-type muscle contraction. In the process of yielding, some of the landing forces are absorbed in order to help prevent injury. However, the key to the explosive movement is to retain as much of the force accumulated on the landing as possible—which means minimizing the amount of flexion in the landing—so you can more powerfully reverse your direction and jump upward. Also, because the energy in the muscle does not last long, the faster you can convert it into upward

153

movement, the greater will be the force pushing you skyward. Thus, by quickly changing the contraction from an eccentric (yielding) to a concentric (overcoming) contraction, the upward jump will be more powerful and higher. In this concentric contraction, the muscle fibers shorten and produce movement, which in this case is extension of the ankle, knee, and hip joints.

As important as these depth jumps are to explosiveness, the Soviets have adapted them a step further in recent years, removing the postlanding leap completely when an athlete is trying to develop eccentric strength. Thus, after jumping off a raised platform, you hold your landing position—essentially trying to stop on a dime as soon as you hit the ground. In this particular exercise, some athletes jump off platforms as high as 6 feet. These, called altitude jumps, aren't recommended for beginners. Before adding them to your exercise program, you need a strong strength base.

Another way of preparing the muscle for an explosive contraction is through isometrics. Using this technique, you would use a maximal or submaximal weight on the body, and hold a position in which the legs are flexed. The position is held for five to six seconds, during which the muscle tension increases greatly. When these seconds have passed, you jump upward as quickly and as forcefully as possible.

The Soviets also use an array of other variations of jumps. You might try some of the following:

1. Step off a box, drop down, and then jump up and over six medicine balls, one by one, that have been laid out in a straight row.

2. Same as above, but jump over three medicine balls, followed by a jump over a low hurdle.

3. Same as above, but after jumping over the three medicine balls, jump straight up for maximum height.

4. Stand between two benches, and then leap up and place one foot on each bench. Jump off, land between the benches, and repeat.

5. Handstand jumps: assume the handstand position (with your feet resting against a wall, if necessary). Then push off with your hands, raising your body upward as high as possible, and returning to a handstand. You'll need assistance to keep your body in a vertical position after each jump.

The throwing of medicine balls and other objects is another effective means of developing arm and total body explosiveness. Begin by assuming the "bottom" throwing position — holding the medicine ball between your legs — to allow the muscles to tense up. Then quickly explode by raising and throwing the object underhand in front, overhead, to the side, and so on.

To utilize the stretch reflex, you should catch medicine balls that have sufficient weight and then immediately repel them. Though the same principles apply here as in depth jumps, throwing involves not only the arms but also the rotational muscles of the trunk. Thus, you develop not only arm strength and speed, but also trunk explosiveness. Keep in mind that when using medicine balls, it is important that they not be too heavy, so that you can go through an effective catch and throw — all in one motion.

Medicine balls, incidentally, can be used to develop leg explosiveness, too, with the help of a friend. Lie on your back with the knees bent and the feet up and facing away. Have your partner throw a ball to you that you can "catch" with your feet in a receiving action, and then quickly repel the ball in an explosive action. Start off with light balls and gradually work up to heavier ones.

Some final thoughts about explosiveness: as I've already suggested, movements of the total body are required for explosiveness in the hands. For example, a baseball pitcher begins his throwing action with a push-off from the leg. In placing his foot forward, he stretches the rotator muscles of the pelvic girdle, which immediately causes a stretch and tension that pull the pelvic girdle around. As the pelvic girdle turns, it stretches the rotational muscles of the trunk, which tenses them and strongly pulls the shoulders around. When this happens, the arm drops down into a cocked position and the shoulder-joint medial rotators are stretched and strongly tensed. They immediately whip forward in the throwing action, at which time the wrist flexors stretch and tense for the final action of wrist flexion and hand pronation. This is the sequence of events involved in all throwing actions that require maximum force or speed. So you can't concentrate on developing only arm explosiveness.

Of course, different sports demand explosiveness of varying degrees. For tennis or racquetball, leg explosiveness is of primary importance, necessary to help you move around the court more quickly. Even so, to execute the tennis serve with maximal speed, some arm explosiveness is needed, too. By contrast, high junipers and long jumpers require relatively little explosiveness in the upper body, but as much leg explosiveness as possible. Basketball and volleyball players use both leg and arm explosiveness in moves like spiking, blocking, rebounding, and ball stealing.

The Soviets also have learned the importance of their athletes doing a lot of sprinting, with particular emphasis on the beginning acceleration. As you might guess, sprinting is an explosive event, and accustoms the body to rapid movement.

If your sport is running — whether competitive or recreational — the importance of developing explosiveness can't be overemphasized. After all, the feet of a high-level sprinter are in contact with the ground for only a fraction of a second at a time. During that instant, the leg muscles must generate forces great enough to propel him or her forward. With the right kinds of training, imagine how much your own performances could improve with increased explosiveness. Figure 13 shows the unique type of apparatus that Soviet athletes have available for just this type of speed strength (as well as strength) training.

As I pointed out in Chapter One, swimmers in the Soviet Union also routinely use speed-strength training. Whereas in the U.S. most coaches believe that larger muscles are the key to success in the pool, the Eastern-bloc swimmers now gradually switch away from strength training to speed-enhancing exercises. Their record-breaking performances in international meets show just how effective this approach has been.

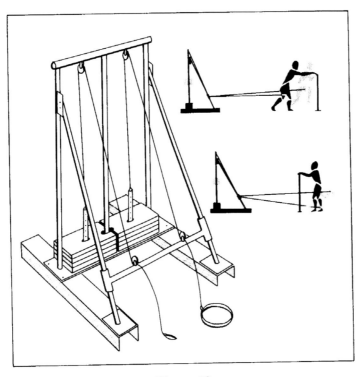

Figure 13.

So just how explosive are you right now? To find out, try performing the vertical jump or the standing long jump. In both cases, the arms as well as the legs are used. The higher you jump, the more explosive you are. And both tests have a high correlation with all sports that require explosive power.

Perhaps surprisingly, the most explosive of all athletes are not runners, jumpers, or swimmers, but weightlifters. Their sport requires not only a great amount of strength, but also enormous speed. In two events—the snatch and the clean and jerk—the lifter is required to raise a maximum amount of weight as quickly as he

157

possibly can, rapidly getting his body under it as he does, which requires tremendous explosiveness in legs, trunk, and arms.

As a result, if you pit a world-class weightlifter against a world-class sprinter, the lifter will almost always accelerate faster in the first 5 to 10 meters of a race. Vasily Alexeyev, the outstanding 350-pound superheavyweight lifter, could run the 100 meters in 11.5 seconds and could do a vertical jump from a standing position of 28 inches. David Rigert, another outstanding Soviet weightlifter who once held world records in two weight divisions, could run 100 meters in 10.4 seconds. Yuri Vardanyan, a world-record middleweight weightlifter for many years, could jump 38 inches vertically, and had a best in the high jump of 7 feet and in the standing long jump of almost 12 feet.

Soviet research into speed-strength training is continuing in some unusual ways. They have developed a variety of sleds and swings for leg explosiveness, as well as harnesses that lift athletes slightly off the ground in order to permit them to run in a lightened state. These methods allow the Soviets to build up speed and explosiveness more quickly than anything yet devised in the U.S.

But using the tools you currently have, you can still reap enormous benefits from a speed training program. In particular, you should emphasize it during the specialized preparatory period. It can be carried over into the competitive period as well. Although it is taxing on the body, the recuperation time is relatively rapid. And as Soviet athletes have consistently proven, the effort certainly has a major payoff, allowing men and women to approach and attain their highest athletic or sports potential.

Chapter 5 Addendum

In the last 30-40 years since its introduction, plyometrics has become a very popular mode of training in the United States. Not only is it now used by all levels of athletes but it is being recommended for fitness buffs. However, the plyometric training being advocated in the athletic and fitness worlds, is not the same as created and advocated by the Russians as described in the original text.

The main reasons for this are misunderstood applications by many "overnight experts" and the introduction of several plyometric texts that presented erroneous information. For example, the books described plyometrics with how jump exercises should be executed, not how true plyometric exercises should be done. Nor did these books give examples of plyometric exercises as described by the Russians.

As a result, all jump exercises have come to be known as plyometric. But they are not. Plyometrics uses jump exercises but all jump exercises are not plyometric. True plyometric exercises are executed in .15-.20 seconds. Many jump exercises as for example, deep squat jumps and jump out of a squat are good for training, but they take over 0.20 sec. to execute. As a result, they cannot be called true plyometric. They fall into the category of jump training which is also of great benefit to the athlete. In general, it precedes plyometric training.

Today, exercises such as skipping rope and easy hopping, skipping and jumping are also considered to be plyometric exercises. They are not. They involve both the eccentric and concentric components but because the execution is so much slower, they are not true plyometric (explosive) exercises. They are of course of benefit; however, they only serve as good beginning or introductory exercises before starting true plyometric exercises that are much more taxing on the body. Thus, do not be misled into thinking that because plyometrics uses different kinds of jumps that all jumps are plyometric.

Also, plyometric exercises do not have to be jump exercises. For example, exercises for the midsection use medicine balls in which you receive and repel the balls as quickly as possible in rotational movements. The same applies to upper body training although you can do jumps with the arms (push-up jumps) as previously described in the main text. If you look closely at some of the diagrams of the equipment used by the Russians in the original text, you can see the various non-jump types of equipment that can be used. This includes sleds, pendulums and swings to elicit the explosive (plyometric) type of muscular contraction.

To help distinguish between the plyometrics that were developed by the Soviets and the plyometrics that are typically done in the U.S., I now use the term shock method as proposed by Dr. Verkhoshansky. As brought out previously, this method is exemplified in the depth jump but its methodology can be used with all exercises. It is the true explosive form of plyometrics that should be used by athletes to develop explosive power.

160

A word must be said here about the sport of weightlifting. As brought out in the original text, weightlifting is an example of a truly explosive (speed-strength) type sport. High level weightlifters are some of the fastest athletes in the world but only for very short distances and for quick acts. Because of this, many strength coaches now utilize weightlifting exercises to develop speed-strength. This is effective for a general transfer of these physical qualities.

However, and this is most important, improvement in sports skills which an athlete must execute in his or her sport does not occur from execution of the weightlifting events! In other words, doing the weightlifting exercises may be effective for developing greater speed and explosiveness, but it will not necessarily transfer to the execution of specific sports skills except for those in which the joint movements duplicate one another.

For example, if you look closely at some of the weightlifting exercises, such as the clean, you can see a direct correspondence to the actions seen in jumping. Thus, this exercise will have a positive transfer to improving jump height. But it does not transfer to greater lateral movement, open field running or movement on a tennis or badminton court. For more information on transfer and the use of various weightlifting exercises, I recommend that you read Transfer of Training by Dr. Anatoly Bondarchuk.

It is also necessary to downplay the over emphasis on maximum strength training for achievement of explosive power. According to the Russian research and even the Russian coaches that I have talked to in the intervening years, this is one of the greatest short comings that they see in American training methods. It seems most strength coaches (especially for football) continue to emphasize the need for greater and greater strength. However, according to the Russians, training for continued increases in strength with maximum weights is a negative, in regard to speed-strength actions. They have shown that world record holders and the greatest Olympic performers do not have the highest results in strength exercises.

This does not negate the need for additional strength. The Russians believe it is very important. One needs additional strength but not by sacrificing speed when it comes to explosive power. It is the excessive strength gains that show up negatively on speed-strength (power) performances. For maximum results in speed-strength events, you need an optimal amount of strength coupled with speed. Speed is the most important factor here because almost all sports skills rely on speed of execution rather than strength of execution. The key is to get the right balance of strength and speed.

Also very important in speed-strength plyometric type exercises is the role of technique. Technique must be coupled with the speed-strength to achieve maximum benefits. As brought out earlier, this is true meaning of conjugate training. You must develop the strength or speed-strength in conjunction with skill execution technique. When this is done, you will have the maximum improvement possible in performance.

For example, in my work with high school level athletes, increases in their 40 times of up to three-four tenths of a second and six inches or more in the vertical jump within a six month period, are not uncommon. At this time much technique work is done not only in skill execution but also in relation to the exercises that are performed, especially in exercises such as the squat, knee drive, pawback, heel raises and true plyometric jumps. For example, developing better running technique will by itself, improve speed as much, if not more than, six or more months of additional general strength training. Even more improvement is seen in quickness once the player learns proper cutting actions.

It is important to emphasize the role of technique in execution of game skills and when performing strength exercises. This is the main priority of the Russians from the very earliest years in the development of athletes. All other factors are considered secondary. This belief and practice is so deeply entrenched that it is taken for granted by Russian coaches and scientists. Because of this, when discussing plyometrics, specialized exercises, skill execution, strength training or other aspects of training, technique is not highlighted—it is assumed that the reader already knows the technique of the sports skill or strength exercise. It is not necessary to constantly reiterate it!

But, as previously mentioned, the teaching and study of technique does not have high priority in the U.S. This includes the teaching of basic and advanced exercises. For example, in regard to execution of strength exercises, I have found that with high school players and even many collegiate players, it usually takes up to 1-2 months to correct (undo) what they learned in the earlier years. Once they begin to execute the exercises correctly, they begin to see great improvement in their performances not only in the strength exercises but in game play.

In regard to athletes who have back or knee problems, I have found that most often it is due to improper technique when executing exercises such as the squat and/or deadlift. With proper technique in these and other strength exercises, especially when they duplicate the technique involved in skill execution, of the plyometric exercise the athlete experiences tremendous improvement in his performance.

If you desire more information on technique of execution of various strength exercises, many of which are prerequisite to doing plyometric exercises, read my book, *Kinesiology of Exercise* and watch the DVD, *Exercise Mastery*. These are the only two sources that go into great detail on how an exercise should be executed and why. These sources bring out all the nuances of the exercise and what will happen when you make changes in grip, stance, etc. or execute the exercise in a different manner.

The Russians are very concerned with movement, i.e. execution of sports skills and exercises rather than simply training muscles. For some reason, we in the U.S., possibly from the popularity of bodybuilding, often emphasize isolating and training individual muscles rather than movements. However, for the best athletic performance, it is necessary to train movements because this is what you must do in game play. This is also key to effective execution of plyometric exercises.

Even the use of exercise machines, as commonly used in many high school and collegiate strength training programs and in general fitness gyms, develops isolated muscles, and retards motor learning. Isolated muscle development makes it more difficult to coordinate the inter- and intra- muscular activity that is critical for effective execution of not only plyometrics but game skills. In addition, doing isolated muscle training, leads to a decrease in the adaptability of the muscles to variations in movement from the basic motor pathway. This is why such exercises are not recommended before doing plyometrics.

For more details on skill execution, especially of the basic skills of running, throwing, jumping, kicking and hitting, it is recommended that you read *Build a Better Athlete*. It is also an excellent source for information on other aspects of training that are very important for an athlete. For more details on plyometrics and illustrations of plyometric exercises be on the lookout for my soon to be released book, *Explosive Plyometrics*.

In conclusion, it is important that you distinguish between true explosive training and exercises that are executed at a relatively slow or moderate rate of speed but still called plyometric. Learn to distinguish jump training from plyometric training by how they are executed. Both play a valuable role. When used in the proper sequence (slow—explosive) they can improve your performance greatly. How the exercise is executed plays the premier role in plyometrics followed by additional strength and speed development.

Chapter 6:

MAXIMIZING YOUR FITNESS POTENTIAL: From Running to Water Sports

In the summer of 1959, an extraordinary track-and-field event took place at the U.S.-U.S.S.R. meet in Philadelphia. On the day of the 10,000-meter run, the weather was vicious, with extremely high temperatures and humidity. In the opening minutes of the race, Robert Soth of the American team got off to an unusually fast start, as if defying the Soviet Union's Hubert Parnakivi to keep up.

Midway through the race, however, the humidity began to take a toll upon Soth. The American became lightheaded and his pace slackened. Then he stumbled, fell to the ground, and fainted on the track as Parnakivi raced by him.

From that point on, Parnakivi had no serious challengers. However, as the Soviet runner approached the finish line and certain victory, he, too, began feeling dizzy and his running stride became disjointed. Exhausted and dehydrated, he nevertheless found a reserve of energy that propelled him through the tape.

Parnakivi had won the race under intolerable conditions, outlasting his top American adversary by several thousand meters. Later, his coach would credit the Soviet runner's rigorous training regimen for his success that day—a training schedule that, by comparison, showed up the preparation of America's athletes as glaringly inferior.

Few can become superathletes like Hubert Parnakivi. But as the Soviet training system becomes increasingly sophisticated, there are techniques and exercises that even the recreational athlete can adopt for his or her specific sport to improve performance and make participating more enjoyable and rewarding.

As you've already learned, the Soviets emphasize getting into excellent all-around shape before concentrating on playing any particular sport. They don't play their sport in order to get in shape (as we tend to do in the U.S.); rather, they get in shape to play their sport.

Once the Soviet athletes have the strong foundation of fitness in areas such as strength, flexibility, agility, and coordination, then they begin focusing on specific exercises that are especially productive for their individual sport. This chapter offers information for many of the most popular American sports — baseball, basketball, cycling, swimming, tennis, and track and field — and you will learn about some of the Soviets' techniques which you can start to utilize.

They have been approaching athletics in this systematic way for years. If you were a boxer in the U.S.S.R., for instance, your trainer would offer more than some tips on defending yourself with your right hand while jabbing with your left. Their studies have dissected the boxing punch in detail and analyzed the precise role that each body part (arms, legs, trunk) plays in its execution. Thus, when they studied the characteristics of a straight right to the head, they discovered that the arm-extension movement accounted for just 24.12 percent of the strength of the punch in Class I (high-level) athletes, compared to 37.42 percent from the trunk's rotational movement and 38.46 percent from the push-off as the back leg extends. Today, with data like these in hand, coaches in the U.S.S.R. have their boxers concentrate much more on improving the strength and speed of the legs and trunk than we do in the West.

Once the Soviets have determined the areas of the body that need specialized attention in a particular sport, they frequently design a piece of exercise equipment (like the one in Figure 14) to help the athlete make the most of his workouts. Coaches in the U.S.S.R. have shown me a variety of devices, such as the highly specialized "sleds" that I mentioned in Chapter Five. These sleds are often used by weightlifters to help develop explosiveness in the legs, working on the particular joint angles that the athlete may be weak in. I've never seen anything like them in the U.S.

With other Soviet devices, the lifter can duplicate the precise movements of the lifts in his events. By adjusting the resistance of these machines, he can accelerate and move as needed during different portions of the lifts. The key here is to duplicate as closely as possible the movements that occur in the sport itself.

Fortunately, you don't have to have equipment as sophisticated as this to make use of what the Soviets have learned. In this chapter you'll find exercises that require either no apparatus at all, or only those machines that you'll find in any American gymnasium or health club.

As earlier chapters have suggested, in many sports, the Soviets work on the entire body to prepare their athletes. Just like the boxers described above, the whole body receives attention in order to maximize performance. If yours is a

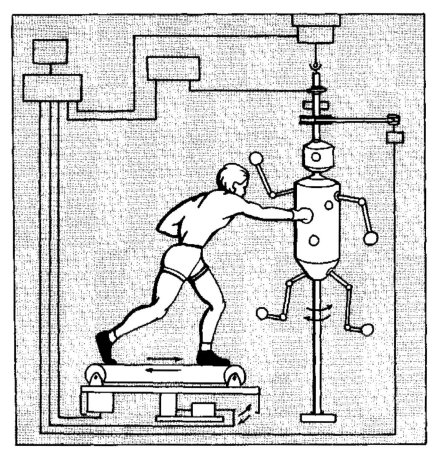

Figure 14

sport where throwing is necessary, for example, you'll need more than just good wrist and arm action. Although some quarterbacks or baseball infielders may be described as "wrist throwers," the wrist, in fact, contributes little. (To prove it, have someone hold your forearm immobile and try to throw a ball; it will travel barely 10 feet.) Throwing involves the legs, the midsection, and the shoulders, as well as the arms and the wrist. It's the whole body that counts.

TRACK AND FIELD

Ralph Mann, a U.S. sports biomechanics researcher, recently published an article that analyzed the running styles of America's elite runners. His conclusions surprised most of our track coaches.

For example, we have assumed for years that to improve sprint speed, the arms have to move faster. But as Dr. Mann's article demonstrated, arm action is not a significant factor in increasing stride rate and other elements that contribute to better performance. Instead, researchers have discovered that the arms "actually hesitate at the dead-end positions; and what we are finding is that the elite athlete is not moving the arms faster, but simply not hesitating as long at the dead-end positions."

Dr. Mann concluded that the key to improvement in the sprints rests in the leg action just before and during contact with the ground. He found that elite runners do not fully extend their legs, and that they run in a more upright position than their slower counterparts. Also, their foot plant tends to be closer to the body's center of gravity — that is, the foot tends to land more underneath the trunk rather than stretching out for extra inches that, in effect, make recovery for the next stride a little more difficult.

Should Dr. Mann's findings have surprised the track-and-field community in the U.S.? In fact, the Soviets had not only known these facts for several years, but had written about them as well. A few years ago, an article appeared in *Soviet Sports Review* in which a sports scientist from the U.S.S.R. reached conclusions identical to those of Dr. Mann. Unfortunately, because this type of research goes largely unnoticed or unheeded in the West, our top runners lag several years behind the Soviets in adopting techniques like these.

So when you sprint, what should you be doing? One valuable suggestion: do not fully extend your leg when pushing off. Even today, many American coaches instruct their athletes that a straight leg is essential to improve running time. But by not allowing your leg to go into full extension, you will save time. It should never be extended at more than an angle of 165 to 170 degrees (180 degrees is completely straight) when the foot is in contact with the ground.

Here are a couple of other tips from the Soviet research labs:

* When you run at a moderate, steady speed, the trunk of your body should be nearly vertical rather than leaning far forward. As speed picks up, however, the trunk angle should increase—but this added lean should come from the spine (at the waist), rather than from flexion at the hip joint. Also, always land on the ball of your foot, not on the heel as some American coaches recommend.

* Hold your head straight while running. Relax the shoulder girdle and the arm muscles, and keep the hands free. Although the fingers should be shaped in the form of a fist, they should not be clenched tightly.

There are a number of specific training exercises that I recommend to improve performance in various track-and-field events. Some require no equipment, and you'll find most of them quite taxing.

Take ankle jumps, for instance. If you want to run with explosiveness, you'll need to work on the ankles, and ankle jumps are among the best exercises that the Soviets have found for this purpose. True, rising up on the toes with weights on your shoulders can build ankle strength; however, I suggest that you rely on jumps to add the explosive element (but only after you've developed enough strength from doing heel raises).

The exercise sounds simple enough. Standing, and keeping your knees as straight as you can, leap as high into the air as possible by fully flexing the ankles. That's all there is to it. However, don't let its simplicity fool you. Most runners, even highly trained ones, have difficulty with this exercise in the beginning. They have become so used to relying on their knee joints that they've never achieved full extension of their ankles. And keeping their knees straight while jumping is initially a struggle.

I suggest that you start by trying to do a set of consecutive ankle jumps. Once you've been able to work your way up to thirty jumps or more, then you can increase the difficulty of the exercise by performing it while holding weights in your hands or a barbell on your shoulders.

One of the benefits of ankle jumps is that they develop resiliency in the ankle muscles. If you find that you have limited ankle flexibility, here is another exercise. Crouch onto your knees, and with your toes pointed behind you, sit down on your heels. This will effectively stretch the area. The more extension you can get in the ankle joints, the more your running will benefit.

Among other ankle exercises, an especially good one is a series of five to ten single-leg and double-leg hops over stationary objects. They can be performed not only with body weight alone, but also with dumbbells in the hands or barbells on the shoulders.

In the Soviet Union, runners who compete at distances of 200 meters or longer are encouraged to develop speed endurance by performing "multijumps" from leg to leg over distances of from 50 to 200 meters. As you might guess, these high-intensity exercises go a long way toward building up endurance.

In the weight room, there are several exercises favored by Soviet sprinters. You've already read about some of them earlier, but let me briefly describe them here:

Squat jumps (Figure 15). With the trunk erect and the legs flexed at the knee joints, jump into the air by rapidly extending both the knees and the ankles.	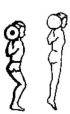 Figure 15
Step-ups with alternate legs (Figure 16). Place the left foot on a raised platform so that a 90-degree angle is formed between the thigh and the lower leg. Then step up on the platform. After lowering yourself, perform the same exercise beginning with the right leg on the raised platform.	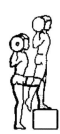 Figure 16

Deep lunge walk (Figure 17). Lunge forward with one leg by rising high on the toes of the back leg. Then bring both legs together and repeat the exercise leading with the opposite leg.	Figure 17
Scissor jumps (Figure 18). With one foot a comfortable distance in front of the other, push off with both feet and ankles, leaping into the air high enough to allow time for your legs to switch positions—that is, your lead foot should land in the rear position, and vice versa.	Figure 18
Jumps from a deep squat (Figure 19). While in a deep squat position, rise quickly on the toes and leap upward. Keep the back erect, and extend the knee and ankle joints fully.	Figure 19
Straight-legged jumps (Figure 20). This is a form of the ankle jumps described above, performed with weights on the shoulders. Leap upward vigorously by extending the ankle joints quickly, keeping movement in the knees as minimal as possible	Figure 20

Running with a high thigh lift (Figure 21). Rapidly alternate legs, fully extending the support leg and lifting the opposite thigh each time, but not higher than the horizontal position. This exercise can be performed either in place or with gradual movement forward.	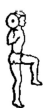 Figure 21

Figure 22 depicts further leg exercises that the Soviets prescribe for their runners. But coaches have the runners go far beyond leg work. They also spend time working on their midsection, for instance, doing abdominal and lower back exercises that will help keep the body erect while competing. The rotational muscles of the midsection must also be strengthened to keep the pelvic girdle from twisting and flailing uncontrollably while running.

To work on this mid-body region, the Soviets have not only found sit-ups to be effective, but also reverse sit-ups and reverse trunk twists. These twisting exercises are critical to stabilize the pelvis.

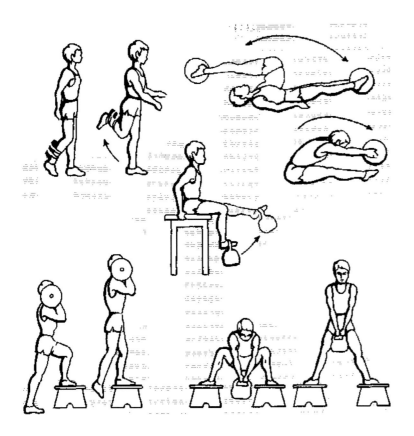

Figure 22. These exercises with weights are commonly used by runners in the Soviet Union.

To perform the reverse trunk twist, lie on your back and place your arms on the floor perpendicular to your body and in line with the shoulders, palms down. Raise your legs directly up until they are perpendicular to the ground (or as close to a 90-degree angle as you can get). Then, while keeping your feet together and your legs straight, lower your legs to the right side, coming as close to touching the ground as possible. Then raise your feet toward the sky again and lower your legs to the left side. Then repeat.

Back raises are important for runners, too. I suggest that you perform them with a partner so the pelvis can be secured, thus concentrating all the action in the lumbar vertebrae of the spine. Lie face down on a table, with your upper body (above the pelvis) extending over the edge. With your partner holding your lower body in place on the table, place your hands on your chest and raise your head and back as high as possible (to a position in which the lumbar spine is slightly arched). Then lower your trunk below the level of the bench. (If no partner is available, you can do this exercise just as well on a Glute-Ham Developer.)

Even though you might think of running as a lower body sport, you can't completely ignore the arms in your training program, particularly if you run long distances. Though the upper body doesn't need explosiveness, the arms and shoulders require muscular strength and endurance to keep the arms moving steadily forward and backward over the miles. So the Soviets have their runners perform exercises that work on the shoulder joints for flexibility and strength, such as dips, in which the body is lowered between two benches (or chairs). And since the aim here is endurance, that means performing a higher number of repetitions—perhaps twenty to thirty at a time.

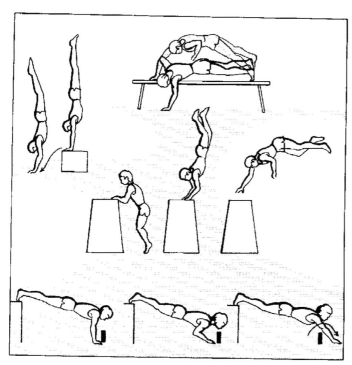

Figure 23. Exercises like these are used by Soviet pole vaulters to build up strength for the push-off from the pole.

All Soviet track-and-field athletes, no matter what their event, spend time working out in the gym. For example, to build strength for the push-off in their event, pole vaulters practice exercises like those illustrated in Figure 23. Pole vaulters also make use of the high bar to simulate some of the movements that they go through during competition. The pulling-up motion they must use as they vault skyward can be duplicated while hanging from the high bar and lifting the legs up until they are above the bar. Vaulters can also perform a variety of twisting maneuvers and "push-offs" from the bar, which again duplicate what is called for in their event.

Special running exercises have also been created for Soviet pole vaulters to help them in their approach runs toward the bar. When you watch vaulters, you can see that their event is made even more complicated by having to approach the bar with their hands "tied up" by holding the pole, and by having to run with the body tilted slightly forward. So the key here is to give athletes a "pole sense" or "feel" while they try to develop a natural stride down the runway.

Thus, in addition to participating in conventional running exercises, the Soviet vaulters perform some or all of the following *while holding the pole:* one-legged jumps, right and left, for 30 to 40 meters; running with a high thigh lift (30 to 50 meters); running with straight legs, emphasizing the planting of the foot (30 to 40 meters); and running with accelerations (30 to 50 meters). Figures 24 through 27 illustrate the unique types of exercises and apparatus the Soviets have developed for their long jumpers, hurdlers, and javelin throwers.

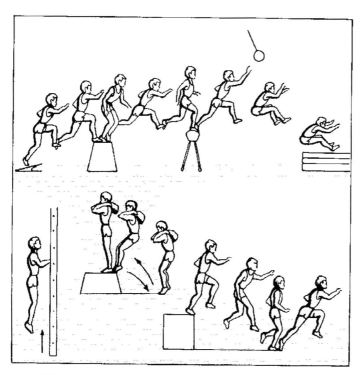

Figure 24. Long jumpers in the Soviet Union rely on exercises like these to develop explosiveness in their event.

CYCLING

Cycling is one of the most popular recreational activities in America, and is an excellent activity for promoting cardiovascular fitness. There are several exercises that I recommend for cyclists, drawn from years of U.S.S.R. sports research.

As you might guess, strong and explosive legs are essential for excelling on the bicycle. Therefore, any number of leg-extension exercises are important for working this area of the body.

I also recommend the glute-ham-gastroc raise described in Chapter Four. It does an excellent job of working on the muscles that are involved in cycling, including the quadriceps, the upper hamstrings, and the gluteus maximus. In fact, it's the only exercise that contracts the hamstring muscles from both ends, permitting full development.

The Soviets also know the importance of the upper torso in competitive cycling. While a leisurely bicycle ride does not require a particularly strong upper body, this region can't be ignored if you take the sport seriously. Particularly when sprinting on the bike, with your trunk properly bent over the bike frame, pulling on the handlebars requires strength. So if you're involved in bicycle racing you'll need strong pulling muscles, which can be achieved with exercises such as seated pulls, rows, and a variety of bicep-strengthening exercises.

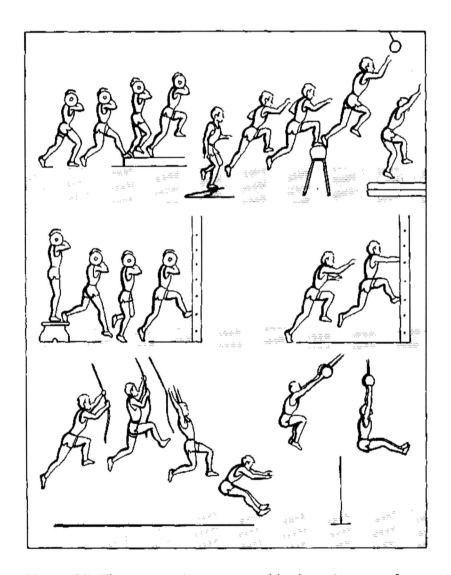

Figure 25. These exercises are used by long jumpers for mastering the technique of both takeoff and flight.

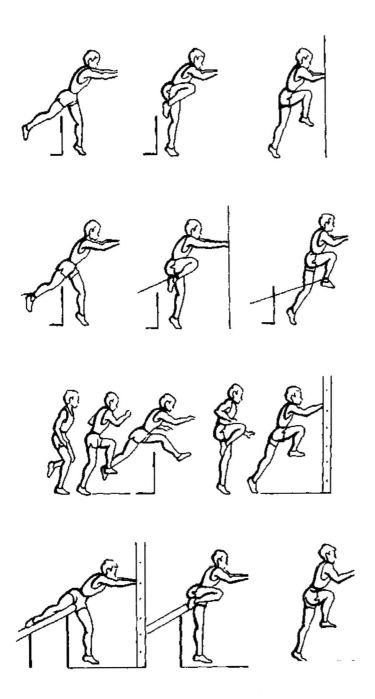

Figure 26. Hurdlers utilize these exercises to perfect the movement of their push-off and swing legs.

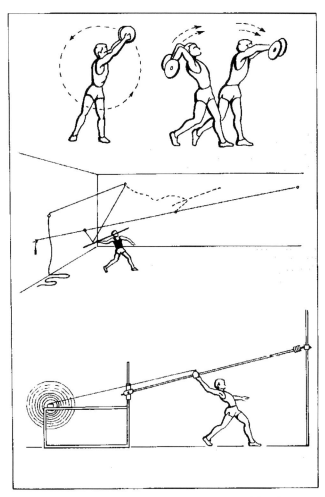

*Figure 27. Javelin throwers use exercises like these
to strengthen the muscles of the arms and
shoulder girdle. They can also take advantage of
special Soviet equipment to train for their event.*

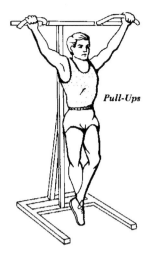

Pull-Ups

Figure 28.

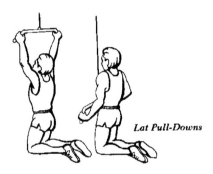

Lat Pull-Downs

Figure 29.

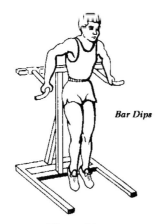

Bar Dips

Figure 30.

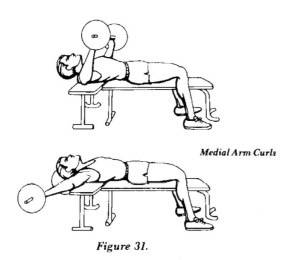

Medial Arm Curls

Figure 31.

SWIMMING

Records in swimming are broken with amazing consistency. Many records have lasted no more than a few weeks—or even days—before being shattered.

Because the competition in the pool is so intense, the world's top swimmers will tell you that they are looking for the smallest of edges. To help their own athletes, the Soviets have developed special weightlifting equipment that duplicates the actual swim stroke, and is used in lieu of the isokinetic machines with which most American swimmers now train. Their researchers have learned that in all swimming strokes, the arm and hand are not driven at a constant rate of speed, but rather move through periods of acceleration and deceleration. Thus, rather than forcing athletes to work their arms at a single speed in the gym, this new Soviet apparatus permits them to reproduce in training the actual movements that occur in the pool.

That isn't all. Training pools in the U.S.S.R. are equipped with machines that can create currents in the water, which the athletes swim into, as a way of maximizing resistance. They even swim while wearing equipment around their waists to further increase resistance, or they use various types of towing devices for the same purpose.

Although much of this equipment is not yet available in the U.S., you can nevertheless make the most of your potential as a swimmer by integrating a variety of accessible exercises into your workouts. To work the upper body, for instance, Soviet research shows that pull-ups, lat pull-downs, bar dips, and medial arm curls are extremely important, duplicating various portions of the pulling action seen in the crawl, breast stroke, butterfly, and back stroke. (See Figures 28 through 31 for pictures of these exercises.) I suggest that you perform them with the grip at various widths to simulate as closely as possible the arm action used in each stroke.

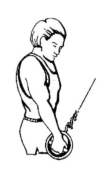

Hand Supination-Pronations

Hand action is extremely important in swimming. Wrist curls and hand supinations-pronations (see Figure 32) are excellent for improving this part of your swimming

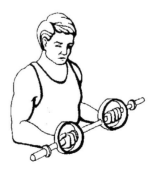

Figure 32.

186

stroke. These exercises are particularly effective when using a device called the Roto-Bar [The Roto-Bar is no longer available], with which you can combine these actions into one movement, and thus more closely duplicate the actions in swimming.

Soviet sports labs have also discovered the importance of combining exercises to approximate the arm strokes in the pool. For instance, begin with the lat pull-down, lowering the bar in front of the body to the chest. Then at the end of the pull, just as action in the shoulder joint ceases, execute medial rotation of the arms.

The lower body also deserves attention in the weight room. In particular, the extensor muscles of the hip, knee, and ankle joints must be worked on. They are needed not only for the leg kicks, but also for the start of each race and the push-off at each turn. Keeping push-off time to a minimum — while maximizing push-off distance and speed — can spell the difference between winning and losing.

The Soviets have found that the most useful exercises for developing the leg muscles of swimmers are heel raises and knee extensions, as well as leg squats in which you rise up on the toes at the end of the upward movement. The leg press is also useful, performed in a seated or flat-on-the-back position. These exercises are shown in Figures 33-36.

More than any other part of the body, the midsection tends to be ignored by American swimmers. This is a mistake. A strong abdomen is important not only to maintain proper body alignment while swimming, but also to enhance the pro-pelling action of various strokes. Soviet research clearly shows that full arm power is impossible unless you have a strong midsection, including abdomen and lower back.

To strengthen the midsection, I suggest that you perform sit-ups, reverse sit-ups, and back raises. It's also important to add twisting movements to these exercises to work on the rotational muscles, which can help keep the hips stabilized in the water. In short, the stronger your abdominals, the faster you'll swim.

Flexibility is also critical for the swimmer, and the Soviets have developed several exercises to work on the shoulder and ankle joints in particular. The following routines should be performed after the body is warmed up, and the stretching on the joints should be increased gradually to prevent stretching the ligaments:

1.   Lie face down, with your chin on the floor and your arms extended straight ahead. Hold a rope or a towel in the hands, and while keeping the arms straight, rotate them backward, up and over your head. At the same time, simulate the leg kick in the crawl stroke. Then return the arms to the beginning position, and repeat. See Figure 37.

2. While lying on your abdomen, bend the left leg at the knee, extending the left foot into the air. Reach back with your right hand and grab the ankle joint of the bent left leg. While arching in the waist, lift the left arm upward. Then return to the original position. After several repetitions, then switch to the opposite arm and leg—that is, grab the right ankle joint with the left hand, and repeat the exercise in the same manner. See Figure 38.

BASKETBALL

Shooting, of course, is the obvious key to success in basketball. But it takes more than just sinking the ball in the hoop to excel in this sport. Maneuverability on the court is just as important. When Soviet basketball players are placed on a training program, their exercises are designed to improve both side and forward movements, as well as quick cutting actions. Side jumps over a bench are widely used for this, as well as forward jumps over benches. Side leg raises are helpful as well.

To maximize explosiveness in the legs, don't overlook depth jumps. The benefits of this exercise will prove particularly useful for jump shots. Try to jump as high as possible, working up to a height of three feet or more.

Also, don't neglect altitude jumps—jumping from a raised platform, which simulate the hard landings that occur repeatedly during a game. In this exercise, you should hold the landing position after reaching the ground. In the process, you'll be landing with an impact of three to ten times your weight, depending on the height from which you jump. The higher you are, the more force will be generated. Even so, to prevent injuries, don't jump from a height of over nine feet, and don't even attempt this exercise until you have built up a strength base.

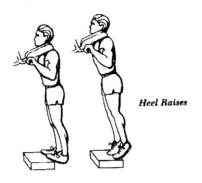

Heel Raises

Figure 33.

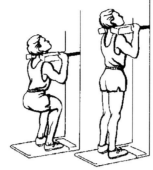

Leg Squat

Figure 35.

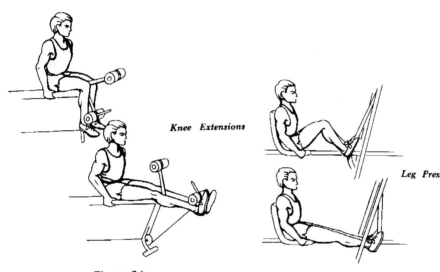

Knee Extensions

Leg Press

Figure 34.

Figure 36.

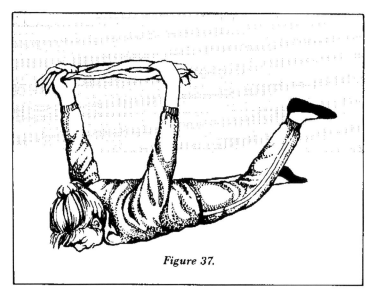

Figure 37.

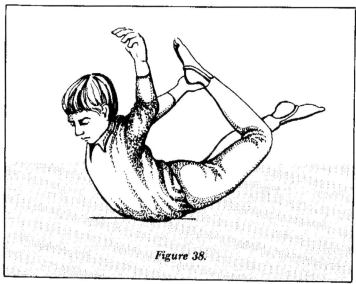

Figure 38.

For variety, the Soviet basketball players also utilize single and double leg hopping with dumbbells in the hands. This exercise can be performed while traveling 10 to 20 yards, or while remaining in place.

As important as it is to work on the legs, the Soviets have not forgotten shooting, either. If you compare the shooting styles of today with those of a decade or two ago, you'll notice that players are compensating for the increased height of their opponents by keeping the elbow up more than ever before, helping the ball sail over the outstretched hands of blockers.

To prepare for making shots like this, overhead triceps extensions and triceps presses are important for building strength. Here are ways that you might work on improving this component of the game:

1. Take a dumbbell in one hand and lift it straight overhead, keeping the elbow close to your head. Then bend your elbow, slowly lowering the weight behind your head until it touches your back. Raise the arm again to the starting position. After fifteen to twenty repetitions, switch hands and do the same with the other arm.

2. With your hands about four to six inches apart—closer than for a normal shoulder press—grasp a barbell and press it overhead. Then slowly lower the weight behind your head, with the elbows kept pointed upward and the arms remaining close to the head. Once the bar is lowered as far as possible—and you've really felt the pull on your triceps—then raise the bar again, extending it over your head to the starting position. (If it's available, use the Roto-Bar during this exercise; it will allow your hand to turn during the extension, and thus to duplicate the shooting action.)

Resiliency is also important in basketball, so the Soviets have their players do a lot of catching and throwing of balls of different weights — a little heavier (to develop strength) and a little lighter (for speed) than a regulation basketball. Particularly as players approach the competitive season, variations in the weight of the balls should be so slight that the players' game technique and coordination are not thrown off by a dramatically different ball. Medicine balls work well here, using the lighter balls to develop more speed, and the heavier ones to work on strength.

Finally, if you play full-court basketball, you will need to develop your cardiovascular endurance. That means long-distance running in the early weeks of training, followed by a combination of slow, fast, and moderate running. The basketball player needs to rely on all three systems — aerobic, anaerobic, and a mix of the two. In particular, try bursting forward and to the side from a slow jog. Basketball players are called upon to do that many times per game.

BASEBALL

Explosiveness is important in nearly every sport, and baseball is no exception. Whether a third baseman is diving to his side for a ground ball, or a runner is accelerating off first base in an attempt to steal second, success depends on explosive ability.

The game of baseball is a truly American sport. But it has recently been introduced in the Soviet Union, largely because it has now become an official Olympic event. Not surprisingly, many of the explosive exercises mentioned earlier have been extremely helpful for the Soviet baseball players, as well as our own athletes when I've recommended them in this country.

Biomechanical analyses show that about 50 percent of the force in throwing and batting comes from trunk and shoulder-girdle rotation. Thus, specialized exercises that work on the rotational muscles have also proven useful— particularly exercises like sit-ups with a twist, back raises with a twist, reverse trunk twists, and Russian twists.

To enhance explosiveness in baseball, spend some time working out with a medicine ball, using a variety of throws. To work on the rotational muscles, for instance, try catching the ball overhead, and then immediately throwing it

193

sidearm or underhand. As you throw, flex in the spine, and get the entire body moving forward into the pitch. As with basketball training, the baseball player can use balls that are lighter or heavier than an actual baseball; keep in mind, however, that during the specialized preparatory period in particular, if the balls weigh considerably more or less than a regulation baseball, your form and technique will be disrupted.

(While watching professional baseball games, you may have noticed that baseball players often swing two or even three bats in the on-deck circle, warming up just before taking their turn at the plate. The Soviets would criticize a technique like this. Two or three bats are too heavy and will throw off the hitter's coordination, even though he may profit from the feeling of lightness once he moves back to a single bat.)

To enhance your throwing potential, try some medial rotation exercises like those that were prescribed for quarterback Todd Marinovich (see Chapter Four). Essentially, you'll be trying to duplicate the baseball throwing motion in the weight room. This might include dumbbell exercises in which the elbow joint is kept at a 90-degree angle, as though you were throwing overhand. Or if you're simulating the throwing of a third baseman or a pitcher, try extending your elbow a little more into a sidearm position. As well as working on strength, you should also be aiming for explosiveness in your throwing motion.

To improve the ability to cut and turn rapidly, baseball players should perform some of the same exercises I suggested in the section on basketball. These include side leg raises (which strengthen the leg muscles), and jumping sideways over a bench (which enhances explosiveness).

RACQUET SPORTS

If you're one of the millions of Americans who regularly play tennis or racquetball, you can benefit from many of the exercises mentioned in the sections on basketball and baseball. As a tennis or racquetball player, you'll constantly be called upon to execute quick side movements, forward movements, and other cutting actions. Thus, more than anything else, concentrate on exercises that enhance the rapid changing of directions.

To develop explosive legs, perform depth jumps and other forms of plyometrics that have already been described. Side-to-side jumps over benches are particularly important. Or set up a maze in which you'll be jumping sideways over small objects while generally traveling in a forward direction.

I also suggest that you work on the rotational muscles mentioned in the section on baseball—specifically, by performing sit-ups with a twist, bent-over trunk twists, back raises with a twist, and Russian twists.

Flexibility is also important in the racquet sports. Fortunately, by playing regularly, your flexibility will improve over the weeks and months. For instance, your first time on the court in many months might find you overstretching to reach the ball, and you will experience soreness in the hip and groin muscles. This occurs because your tissues have shortened during your layoff, restricting the flexibility in your joints. In time, however, you'll gradually regain flexibility as you continue to play, and soon you should be playing pain-free. You can speed up the process by doing some stretching exercises before beginning to play.

VOLLEYBALL

You can't be a well-rounded volleyball player unless you can jump. Proper spiking and blocking rely on your ability to soar above the top of the net. Consequently, the exercises in the basketball section designed to enhance your leaping ability will be particularly helpful to your volleyball game.

In addition to techniques like depth jumps, the Soviets have developed other exercises that have been quite useful for their national volleyball team (as well as for athletes from many other sports). For instance:

1. Push forward and upward with your left leg, land on your right, and then as soon as your left leg is brought even with the right, immediately take off energetically with both legs. This final jump should be accompanied by arched arm movements that bring the arms overhead, reaching for the sky. The exercise should be one continuous movement; any stopping impairs your ability to get full benefit from it. (See Figure 39.)

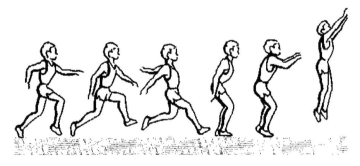

Figure 39.

2. Stand with the right side of your body alongside an exercise bench. Place your right leg on the bench, leaving your left on the floor. Then, by extending your right leg, leap skyward, accompanied by a circular movement of the arms in an upward direction. Land with your right leg back on the bench, and the left on the floor. During this exercise, the left leg

should be used only to maintain balance and coordination of movement. After ten jumps, move to the other side of the bench and take off with the left leg for ten repetitions. (See Figure 40.)

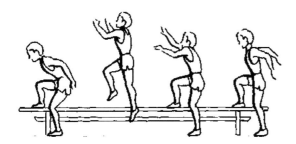

Figure 40

3. Jump with both legs on a bench, a table, a rolled up mat, or another piece of equipment. After jumping down, turn around and repeat immediately with as little a pause as possible. Do five to ten repetitions. The height of the equipment depends on your own ability, but you should try to increase it over time. (See Figure 41.)

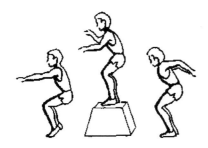

Figure 41.

4. This exercise requires the assistance of a teammate. Have him or her pass the ball to you in a high set, as if you were about to spike it. But instead of hitting the ball, jump up and catch it, leaping as high as possible with both arms. Do five to eight consecutive repetitions. (See Figure 42.)

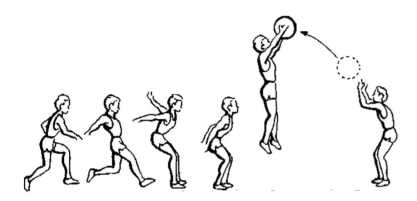

Figure 42.

Using exercises like these, Soviet volleyball players have increased their leaping ability by 3 to 4 inches in a single season—an achievement that is particularly remarkable when that kind of gradual improvement is seen repeatedly, year after year, over the career of a single athlete.

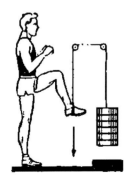

Example 1. Leg Extension

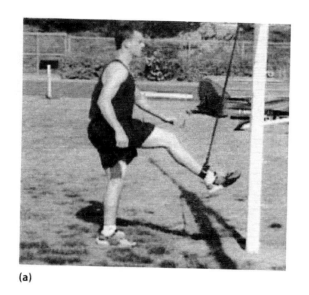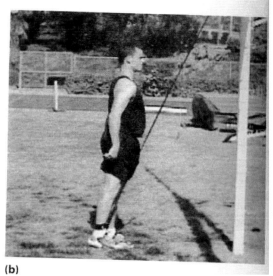

(a) (b)

Example 2. Pawback with Active Cords

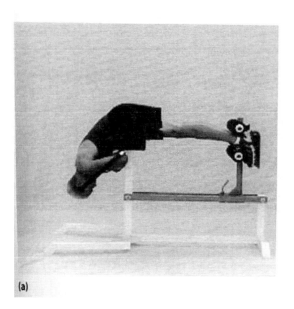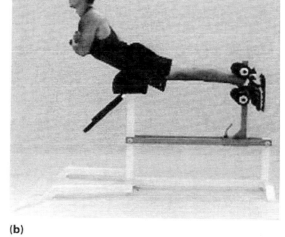

(a) (b)

Example 3. Back Raise

Chapter 6 Addendum

The information presented in this chapter needs a little updating especially in regard to the technique involved in the different events and the specialized strength and explosive exercises that duplicate execution of the sports skills. Because of the complex details and amount of information available, I have incorporated much of the Russian information together with my own research and practical experiences into several books.

For example, in *Explosive Running*, there is extensive coverage of the biomechanics (technique) when running at different speeds and the kinesiology of running (the muscle and joint actions and the coordination between them). In addition, active stretches specific to running, correction of common running errors through specialized strength exercises and chapters devoted to specialized strength and explosive exercises that duplicate the neuro-muscular pathways are presented in this book. Thus, for anyone interested in running, regardless of whether you are a track athlete or run in your sport, this book is a great learning and training source.

Many of the exercises described in the book can be done at different rates of execution. When done at a moderate rate they are excellent exercises for strength for all levels of performers. However, when the objective is to increase speed, the exercises are done more explosively--as quickly as possible. For example, in the touchdown in running, as soon as the foot makes contact with the ground, you absorb some of the landing forces but withstand most of the landing forces in order to then immediately return them in the forward push-off. To duplicate this action in the ankle joint extension you should do ankle jumps. The quicker the jump is executed, the higher you will go in the jump and the more you will develop the quick muscle reaction. This action can then be transferred to sprinting and even long distance running if executed at a slightly slower rate with jump training. Note that ankle jumps are the same as straight legged jumps.

Such explosive execution as needed in sprinting, constitutes a true explosive exercise for which most of the described exercises are well suited. To ensure that the exercises are explosive, they must be executed in approximately 0.15-0.2 seconds. This is the amount of time taken for the landing and takeoff. Recall that in running, the foot is in contact with the ground for all of 0.1 sec.--0.05 sec. for the landing and 0.05 sec. for the takeoff. However, it is impossible to duplicate a takeoff in this amount of time artificially. You must be running at top speed in order to illicit this quick contraction. But, doing the explosive exercises as mentioned are still of great benefit as they improve your ability to decrease the actual amount of ground contact time in the all-out run.

In regard to the exercises in the original text, the deep lunge walk is still a good exercise. However, the classic (Russian) lunge done with Active Cords is superior. Because of the resistance of the cords, you duplicate more of the true running stride in the movement. Emphasis should be on ankle joint extension, the key action involved in the pushoff. You duplicate this with an explosive (leaping) lunge. The deep lunge walk would be a good preparatory exercise especially in GPP.

Running with a high thigh lift, is a good exercise during the GPP period, but is not recommended for higher level runners during SPP. As brought out, the key action in sprinting is to drive the thigh forward, not upward. Thus, this exercise can teach bad habits and not improve your running speed--or agility. The best exercise to develop the hip flexors as they work in running, is the knee drive with Active Cords.

In regard to the midsection abdominal and lower back exercises, for more information on execution of each of these exercises, it is recommended that you read *Kinesiology of Exercise*. It goes into great detail on exercise execution, the muscles involved, what happens when you make any changes or deviations in the execution, and for which sports they are best suited. The book is well illustrative with photographs of the exercise and additional drawings of the muscles.

As you study each of these different exercises, note that they apply not only to running and other track and field events, but also to other sports. For example, gymnasts can use many of these exercises in their free exercise and vaulting events. They can also be used successfully by football, baseball, basketball, hockey and other players to improve strength, speed and quickness.

Cycling and Swimming

For cycling, the information is still basically the same. However, additional specialized exercises for cycling can be developed. There is also a need for more specialized work on duplicating race conditions with more work done on prevention of lower back problems. Also important are additional strength and speed-strength exercises to increase leg power for the sprints and speed endurance for the longer distances.

For example, a sample exercise for strength of the hip extensors would be execution with the use of weights as shown in figure 43. In figure 44 you can see basically the same exercise done with Active cords. Instead of having the leg straight as shown in figure 44 the exercise can be done with a bent knee and the attachment can be at the lower thigh. When done with Active cords the exercise can also be done explosively to develop the power needed in the sprints. By decreasing the resistance and increasing the repetitions and executing the exercise at a slower rate of speed to duplicate race speed, you can develop the speed endurance needed for the race. Similar exercises can be done for the leg (knee) extension.

To strengthen the lower back the Russian use the back raise, which is best done on a Glute-Ham Developer, or on a sturdy table with someone holding your legs down. This is the only exercise that strengthens the lower back muscles through the full range of motion. It is by far the best low back exercise for cyclists and other athletes. See figures 45 A and B.

Swimming can be improved even more so today with the use of more specialized exercises. Coaches should get more involved in analyzing swim technique and then developing exercises that duplicate what occurs in different portions of the swim stroke. For example, duplicating the freestyle pull is already fairly well established although many exercises are not differentiated according to the phase of the pull. For example, pulling back with a bent arm from slightly above the shoulders to slightly below the shoulders and pulling back with the elbow pointed down (shoulder joint extension) or to the side (shoulder joint adduction).

There are also key exercises for the forearm and hand (pronation/supination) that can be executed with the strength bar with the arm in front of the body in the same position as when swimming. This positioning is necessary as there may also be some medial shoulder joint rotation occurring at the same time. There are also wrist flexion actions that can be strengthened at the end of the pull phase as well as the medial shoulder joint rotation that occurs in not only the freestyle but in the breaststroke, butterfly and backstroke. Exercises can be developed for each of these different aspects with the use of Active Cords, the strength bar and other pieces of equipment. Also useful for some swimmers is strengthening of the fingers and wrists with the ExerRings to hold hand position during the pull.

Basketball

I have used much of the information gleaned from the Russians in the training of basketball players. When technique is analyzed and improved, not only in shooting, but cutting actions, jumping, running and sprinting, players are able to improve their abilities greatly. Because of the great detail involved in each of the exercises for each of these different skills, I compiled this information in *Explosive Basketball Training*. It can greatly benefit anyone interested in this sport and how to improve most any aspect of play.

All too often coaches use only ball drills and conditioning exercises to improve performance. However, these are a far cry from what could be done. Understand that ball drills are only as effective as the skill level of the player will allow. If the player doesn't have the skills developed to a sufficiently high level, he will not be able to execute the drills as effectively as possible nor will he or she get the improvement hoped for.

Even basketball shooting has evolved more in the past 21 years. If you look at high level players today you will see that the shooting action is basically executed with elbow extension and wrist flexion. Novices, youngsters and most women still use the push pattern in which they utilize the shoulder, elbow and wrist joints to get enough force to propel the ball to the basket. The more advanced technique, however, has evolved in order to get the ball even higher, out of reach of the opposing player.

To train for this new technique, players should do specialized exercises as described in the original text to develop the feel and the strength needed for the actions. For example, single arm overhead elbow extension. This is an excellent exercise to teach the player to keep the elbow up high and then execute elbow extension--the key action in shooting the ball. Doing exercises for the wrist action are also important. This includes not only basic strength exercises such as the wrist curl, but also explosive wrist flexion done with a small weighted ball.

Additional special exercises commonly used in sprinting can also be used to improve running, acceleration and taking the first step. When players are able to execute cutting actions sharply and quickly as described in *Explosive Basketball Training*, they will see their quickness on the court improve up to 50%.

Baseball

Baseball is not a popular sport in Russia. Even though it is the national U.S. sport it should be noted that on the professional level, close to 50% of the players are from foreign countries. This is indicative of the fact that the U.S. is not developing the talent that it presently has. As brought out previously, one of the most startling discoveries by the Russian coaches after seeing what takes place in the United States, is that we do a very poor job of developing the talent that we have. According to them, if we were to do a better job of developing our talent, the rest of the world would have a very hard time keeping up with us.

What is glaringly absent in baseball is the use of high shutter speed visual video analyses of pitching and hitting actions. Teams still rely on pitching or hitting coaches to look at the players to figure out what they are doing instead of specialists. However, as we know from biomechanices, it is impossible for the eye to see what happens in these actions because they occur too quickly.

There should also be analyses of the players' running and acceleration capabilities to increase running speed and base stealing. These skills are in great need of improvement since it is rare to find players with effective technique. Such analyses are also needed before one can prescribe specialized exercises to improve or correct technique and to prevent injury.

It appears that most professional and even high level players in the minor leagues and collegiate levels have for the most part, effective abilities that enable them to play well even though they may lag behind in specific physical abilities or technique. But, most players appear to come into spring training out of shape and spend spring training and the early part of the season getting in shape merely to play on the same level that they did the previous year. There is no scientific system or periodization plan (especially block periodization) for these players to improve their performance or even to be able to play consistently on a high level for the entire season. For more information in these areas it is recommended that you read, *SPORTS: Is it all B.S.?* and the many baseball (and other sports) articles that appear on the dryessis.com sports training blog site.

Racket sports

If you follow tennis, you will notice that there are many top Russian women and several top men players in professional tennis. This is not due to chance alone. The training that many of these players had and presently do allow them to develop to a higher level than their American counterparts. In fact, it does not appear that there are any up and coming American men or women who will soon be stepping into or dominating the top 5 of the world's best. For example, there wasn't a single male player remaining after the third round in Wimbledon in 2008. Although the Williams sisters were victorious, it was the first time in many years and they continually have injuries.

The lack of top players, especially when we see how many top competitive players there are from other countries, is indicative of the poor player development programs in tennis. Until the USTA and other responsible organizations look into advanced techniques as outlined in this book and elsewhere, player development will continue on a sub-par level. In the meantime, many European (and Asian) countries are incorporating these principles and developing players superior to American talent. As mentioned with baseball, block training, visual biomechanical analyses and incorporation of specialized strength and explosive straining can go a long way to developing the talent.

For anyone interested in additional tennis training methods, some of which are based on the Russian system and exercises, it is recommended that you study the CD, *Explosive Tennis: The Forehand* and *Explosive Tennis: The Backhand.*

Volleyball

Since the time of writing the original text, U.S. volleyball has improved greatly. This is due not only to a wider selection of players but also to superior training methods, many of which are based on concepts used by the Russians. One area that can still use additional improvement is in the use of more specialized strength exercises.

For example, in my work with high level professional volleyball players, I have devised many exercises that duplicate some of the key skills and functions that they must execute. This includes doing exercises such as front arm pull downs beginning with an arched back to duplicate what occurs in blocking, the knee drive for a quicker first step and acceleration, single arm overhead elbow extension and pronation for spiking, the Russian twist for greater truck rotation in the spike and digging balls, executing forward or backward movements out of a jump landing and so on.

These were some of the exercises that I created for Dianne Denechochea, a professional beach volleyball player. To create these exercises I first filmed her during competitive play to see where she was lacking or needed enhancement. We discussed the various movements and then the exercises followed. In addition, single leg exercises were done to duplicate many movements that took place on one leg. Jumping in different directions on one leg as sometimes occurs during game play was something that she and other athletes had never before experienced. This training was responsible for her becoming one of the best tour players.

Chapter 7:
The Soviet Science of
Sports Psychology

How do basketball players who sink only 60 percent of their foul shots one season improve their performance to 85 percent the next? How can a high jumper who had tried for years to break the 7-foot barrier suddenly be able to soar over it, time after time? How does a volleyball player who had always felt intimidated at the net remarkably change into an aggressive blocker and spiker almost overnight?

As you might assume, physical and technical preparation on the field are critical for each of these high-achieving performers. But what about the athlete who is in superb physical shape, yet still has not achieved the results of which he or she seems capable? For these (and all other) athletes, there is a growing recognition that psychological—not just physical— factors play an important role in sports excellence. A physically superior athlete may not have the edge over *a* less-talented opponent, if that opponent is better prepared psychologically and emotionally for competition.

The ancient Greeks actually recognized the value of sports psychology over two thousand years ago. If a Greek runner, for instance, turned pale just before his event, he was not allowed to compete, since his pallor was considered a sign of fear. The Greeks also prescribed soothing music for excitable athletes just before competition.

Today, some American coaches have started to incorporate sports psychology into the training programs of their athletes. However, in most of -these cases, psychological techniques are applied rather randomly and experimentally, and mainly to prepare an athlete for a particular upcoming meet or game. Unfortunately, by then, the athlete has in all likelihood already developed psychological difficulties related to his or her sport.

But in the U.S.S.R., things are different. The Soviets were the innovators of modern practical sports psychology and have been refining it for decades. It is now considered an important part *of every* athlete's training, not just those with problems or those at the top level. In fact, entire textbooks have been written on the psychological preparation for each of a number of major sports—hockey, basketball, volleyball, shooting (archery/guns), and so on.

Their sports scientists are rapidly learning to detect and neutralize psychological factors that can interfere with an athlete's performance. Whether it's fear, anxiety or pregame excitement, a strained state of mind can keep an athlete from competing up to potential. Researchers have become quite sensitive to the disruptive influence that fear can have upon sports performance. Studies show that athletes are often intimidated not only by their opponents, or the height of the bar that they must jump over, or the barbell they must lift. Some also are afraid of the stopwatch, the starting blocks, the crowd, and other influences that, at first glance, might not seem to be important.

A number of approaches not known in the U.S. have been developed in the U.S.S.R. to help coaches evaluate and overcome athletes' fears. For instance, imagine your own coach having access to a transducer for measuring electrical resistance of the skin. Or an instrument for determining the level of emotional excitement. Or a device for analyzing the potential of the cortex of the brain to concentrate on the competition at hand, which can vary depending on your fatigue levels.

In the U.S., top athletes rarely have more than one or two meetings with a sports psychologist, while their peers in the U.S.S.R. are immersed in an array of programs. There, athletes are placed on a six-month-long psychological training schedule to develop proper mental attitudes. Thereafter, they spend at least ten to fifteen minutes of every training day in psychological preparation. It's a year-round regimen, as much a part of training and competition as warmup exercises.

The reason that Soviet sports scientists have decided that psychological training is so important is clear. No matter what level of sports you've competed in—high school, college, or professional—you're familiar with the stress and tension that can be part of that experience. Soviet studies show that one of every three athletes performs below his or her capabilities for no reason other than this stress.

However, you can utilize specific psychological techniques that can help ease much of that anxiety. Through various mental exercises that can help manage breathing and concentration, for example, you can improve your performance on the athletic field. The Soviets have learned that with psychological preparation, you can create coolness under pressure, self-confidence, and a fighting spirit. You can focus on the competition itself, entering an almost hypnotic state in which crowd noise all but vanishes and sensations of pain often disappear.

Before competing, athletes in the U.S.S.R. are prepared psychologically so that they:

* know precisely what they will be called upon to do in the upcoming event;

* have a complete understanding of their body's capabilities that particular day, and confidence in their ability to perform to their maximum potential;

* know the strengths and weaknesses of their opponents, and have actually trained against teammates who have re-created exactly how that opponent is likely to perform;

* can successfully combat negative emotions that may be provoked by the competition; and

* are fully aware of the conditions of the competition that day, including weather and lighting. In fact, weeks before competition, coaches will travel to the site of the event to determine where the lights are located, where the crowd sits, and what the noise levels are likely to be; and this entire competitive environment will be duplicated as closely as possible during training.

It is worth discussing some of the more popular — and successful — psychological techniques that have been developed, streamlined, and implemented behind the Iron Curtain. Auto-conditioning (also called self-regulation or autogenic training), for instance, has been developed in the U.S.S.R. since 1957, but has only recently been making some inroads in the West. Essentially, auto-conditioning is a means of not only relieving stress, but also permitting the athlete to harness that stress and use it in a *positive* way.

Dr. Gregory Raiport, who has conducted sports psychology research in the Soviet Union, has described auto-conditioning as a means of returning "control of the athlete's body back to the athlete — which is, of course, where it belongs." Others have compared it to self-hypnosis, in which the individual learns to control everything from heart rate to blood pressure. In essence, it is an active means of self-regulating involuntary bodily functions.

Here's how this technique works. An athlete, sitting in a chair, is given commands like "feel cold," "feel heat," or "work up a sweat." The first time this is tried, not much is likely to happen. But after several sessions of ten to fifteen minutes each, and as athletes become more familiar with feedback from their own bodies, they are amazed at how effective the technique can become.

Eventually, rather than allowing stress to interfere with their performance, they can capture that energy and utilize it in a beneficial way — for instance, by learning to secrete more adrenaline (an energy-providing hormone) into the bloodstream whenever they require an extra boost. To elevate adrenaline levels, the athlete will focus on thoughts like "I'm not afraid of my opponent . . . I'm going to beat this guy . . . I'm better than he is ... I'm going to fight and win." After considerable practice, this technique can literally get the adrenaline pumping. In much the same way, commands such as "everything is okay" (to calm oneself) or "you're doing wonderfully" (to build self-confidence) have contributed positively to an athlete's performance.

The Soviets generally recommend that their athletes schedule these sessions before sleep at night and upon waking in the morning. The morning session is designed to instill positive messages related to the training activities of that day. The evening session is directed primarily at eradicating unfavorable experiences or impressions that may have occurred earlier in the day. It should also serve to encourage a quiet night's sleep with full restoration, both physically and psychologically.

For auto-suggestion techniques like these to be effective, the athlete must first be thoroughly relaxed. For this reason, all Soviet athletes must learn relaxation training. In essence, they are taught to achieve a feeling of progressive warmth and relaxation in the muscles of their legs, pelvic girdle, spine, abdomen, chest, arms, neck, and face. This relaxation is important for both intramuscular and intermuscular coordination, and is often achieved by tensing (or maximally contracting) each muscle group, one by one, and then releasing that tension (or maximally relaxing). They also learn to slow down their breathing and retard their heart rate. Only then are they ready to instill suggestions that can stimulate confidence and positive attitudes.

They might begin by simply thinking, "I quiet myself," and "I breathe deeply and quietly." The Soviets suggest that the word "I" should be carried out on the inhalation, and "quiet myself on the exhalation. Then some positive statements are recited silently:

* I feel myself quiet and assured.
* I am prepared to struggle for victory.
* I am thoroughly ready to compete.
* I am full of strength and energy.
* I feel light and free.

Over time, individuals can so perfect their ability to relax that they can enter this state in a matter of seconds, simply by willing themselves into it. Even in the midst of competition, they can relax on command, thus economizing and conserving their energy.

I have talked to many Soviet athletes who have described the benefits they've received from this instant relaxation. Imagine the pole vaulter, for instance, who is given three attempts at a particular height, and who, over the course of a meet, may vault a dozen or more times. Between tries, it's important for him to avoid tightening or tensing up before his next attempt. By learning to relax on command, he can remain in peak form for his next vault.

Relaxation techniques like these are well-known in the U.S., of course, but they are rarely used systematically in athletic training.

As effective as approaches like this can be, the Soviets also continue to rely on more traditional psychological aids such as hypnosis. In the initial session with an athlete, the Soviet sports hypnotist explains what hypnosis is and what it can accomplish, its safety, and its similarities to natural sleep. The athletes are also told that under hypnosis, they can build self-confidence, overcome fears, and recover from fatigue more rapidly.

Then they lie down, close their eyes and calm themselves. Breathing becomes easy. They are told to feel themself wanting to sleep . . . more and more . . . wanting to sleep.

Short hypnotic sessions last from two to fifteen minutes, but longer ones can go for up to eight hours or more. During this time, the athlete is instilled with a number of appropriate suggestions. For instance: "Your muscles are well-rested . . . fatigue has completely gone away ... an enormous increase in strength has come to you."

There are other useful techniques routinely used behind the Iron Curtain. Mental rehearsal or visualization is one of them. Even if you're not utilizing the Soviets' highly refined version of this approach, you probably apply it on some level — perhaps by daydreaming about the serve that sped by your opponent in last week's game, or by picturing the day you crossed the finish line ahead of another runner in the 100-meter dash when she or he was supposed to win in a breeze.

At its best, visualization is a real skill. It involves creating a "screen" in your mind's eye and consciously fashioning images that can have a positive impact. More than anyone else, the Soviets have formalized this technique and made it a routine part of their training programs.

Here's an approach you can try that will give you a sense of what the Soviets are doing with visualization:

Sit in a comfortable place, with your legs and arms uncrossed. After assuming a relaxed position, close your eyes and recall a particular athletic performance in which you excelled. Perhaps it was a superb game of tennis or an outstanding 5-kilometer run. Visualize the scene as vividly as possible. Where was it? Indoors or out? What time of day? What was the weather like? What could you see and hear?

Picture yourself immediately before performing. What were you wearing? How did you prepare yourself in the moments before competition? When the activity began, how did you use your arms and legs? As it continued, what exactly did you do to get to the finish line? What were the bodily sensations that you experienced? What were you thinking about at the time? What were your emotional feelings during and after the event?

The Soviets have discovered that when such images are visualized just before competition, they can help an athlete overcome pregame jitters, replacing anxious thoughts with mental pictures of success. Rather than concentrating on negative pictures that can weaken performance, the athlete can direct attention to produce positive results.

Intriguingly, Soviet research shows that as you vividly imagine yourself competing and your body performing to perfection, this activity actually sends subtle nervous impulses from the brain to the muscles involved in that activity. As you picture yourself shooting one successful free throw after another, actual learning is going on, and you are leaving an imprint of precisely how your body movements should be organized in order to sink shot after shot. In this process— called ideomotor training—you are putting your brain and your muscles through their paces. Although any overt body movement is negligible, you are nevertheless preparing yourself for competition. For this reason, your images should be as vivid, detailed, and accurate as possible; if you visualize errors in your form, for example, they may ultimately be translated into mistakes on the playing field.

To get the most out of this exercise, you should proceed through the mental rehearsal at the same speed at which the event itself actually took place. Thus, if you run the 100-meter dash in 10.5 seconds, you should visualize it at that speed; if you slow it down in your mind's eye, you'll in essence be rehearsing or practicing it—and programming your body—at that slower speed.

As a general rule, you should practice these mental exercises daily, and particularly in the minutes immediately preceding competition. Relive every aspect of your success, and really *feel* it as you do. Let it sink into your psyche and your body, detail by detail.

Thus, swimmers should vividly picture themselves approaching the pool, removing their sweats, being introduced to the crowd, climbing onto the starting platform, leaping forward at the sound of the gun, swimming with perfect strokes, making the turns flawlessly, and so on.

Here are portions of a visualization exercise that a Soviet sports coach regularly uses with his world-class swimmers when they are seated in a relaxed position with their eyes closed:

Imagine that you are in a group of swimmers awaiting the start of the afternoon's competition. You are a little nervous, but less than usual. You have done a lot of preparatory work, and now the time has come for you to show just what you are capable of. Today, everyone is seeing a new high-class swimmer, capable of swimming the 400-meter freestyle in less than 3 minutes 50 seconds. You know that this can be a routine time for you. You can do it on any occasion, under any conditions. You are an athlete who has already swum at this speed, and you are ready for a new personal record. You are confident of this and now everyone will see it. ...

Now your heat is being called to the start. You are heading for the starting blocks. In your body, there is slight excitement and nervousness. You stop opposite your starting block. You warm up. Your whole body is warm and supple. Your arms turn easily in the joints. Movements are easy.

At the first whistle, don't hurry to start undressing. Place your clothes neatly on the back of the chair. At the second whistle, stay at the back edge of the starting block. Lean forward at the next whistle.

The gun goes off, and you fly off like a bullet. You swim the first two strokes without breathing. Movements are easy. Your arms have a good feel for the water. You are swimming unbelievably easily, without any effort. A feeling of enormous power appears. Now you are really flying; you are flying over the water. The sight is beautiful. Your movements are economical and graceful. Looking at you, spectators become enthusiastic, and this gives you strength. You are easily staying up with the leading group. You are swimming easily, with delight. Your movements bring you joy. . . .

Soviet psychologists are convinced of the importance of imaging the emotions involved in the event, and not just the satisfaction and elation that come when competition is over. They believe that feelings from beginning to end — from walking onto the playing field before the game to leaving for the locker room when it's all over — should be integrated into the process.

The athletes in the U.S.S.R. also use a number of other psychological techniques in their training schedules and competitive regimens. For instance, many coaches in the U.S.S.R. are strong believers in the "act as if" technique. Using this method, they have their athletes act a part, *pretending* that they have qualities which may be desirable but which they really don't possess.

Let's assume that you are highly anxious just before a major track meet. Rather than exhibiting that tension and uneasiness externally, the Soviets would recommend that through your movements and expressions, you suggest a state of cheerfulness and confidence. Act the part, they say. As you do, you'll actually start to feel more positive. And in the process, you just might intimidate your opponent.

I recall an East German shot-putter who could scare you into defeat just with the aura he projected. By the things he said and the mean way he looked at you, he made any competitor feel inferior. It was all part of his psychological game, and it gave him an edge that helped him win one meet after another.

Music is another psychological tool used by Eastern-bloc athletes, with research showing that it can affect one's emotional state by producing positive feelings and attitudes. Specialized massage techniques are also frequently used as a way of quieting and calming an athlete. Even colors have been found to influence athletes in different ways — green relaxes while red creates anxiety and excitation.

Some American athletes now comprehend the importance of sports psychology. Bruce Jenner demonstrated his appreciation for mental techniques when he recently said, "At the Olympic level, the physical capabilities of athletes are all very close. . . . Athletic competition at this level is eighty percent mental challenge and twenty percent physical challenge."

Jack Nicklaus has written, "I never hit a shot, not even in practice, without having a very sharp, in-focus picture of it in my head. It's like a color movie. First I 'see' the ball where I want it to finish, nice and white and sitting up high on the bright green grass. Then the scene quickly changes and I 'see' the ball going there: its path, trajectory and shape, even its behavior on landing. Then there is sort of a fadeout, and the next scene shows me making the kind of swing that will turn the previous images into reality."

Approaches like this are commonplace in the U.S.S.R. As much as anything else, these techniques prepare their athletes so well for competition that they don't need a coach to lean on for support at all times. In one of my trips I stayed at the home of a Soviet coach in Minsk, who brought this point home to me vividly.

One afternoon this coach told me, "Mike, congratulate me. I just got the word that one of my top athletes won in his event at a big meet in Moscow, which means that I've turned out enough winners to satisfy the requirements to keep my job." He explained to me that in the U.S.S.R., coaches are evaluated by how many winners they produce, and if their elite athletes don't perform up to expectations, their own jobs may be in jeopardy.

I was happy for my friend, but at the same time surprised. "What do you mean that one of your top athletes just won?" I asked. "You're here in Minsk. What was he doing in Moscow without you?" A puzzled look came over his face. "What did he need me for?" he asked. "He's a big boy. He can handle himself at a major meet."

It sunk in. Because of the excellent psychological and physical training that the U.S.S.R. puts its athletes through, they can go to meets without needing to have a coach there to hold their hands. They are taught to be in command, and to be responsible enough to care for themselves, from minor meets to major international events. By contrast, American coaches are routinely on the sidelines when their athletes compete,

Obviously the Soviets don't yet have all the answers. Although intensive research into sports psychology is ongoing in the U.S.S.R., this is an area where there is still a lot to learn. Even so, just by utilizing the approaches that have already been developed behind the Iron Curtain, you may be able to achieve that advantage you've been seeking in your own competitive world. If you want to improve your performance, I suggest that you give these techniques a try.

Chapter 7 Addendum

Very little if anything can be added to this chapter at this time. Suffice it to say that the Russians use sports psychology to a great extent to train the athlete rather than using it only as a means of helping to alleviate anxiety or stress. In other words the psychology is used to train the athlete to have a particular frame of mind and to be able to execute in a certain way, express certain emotions, to utilize the emotions and thought processes, etc. in the most productive and effective manner. For example, I have seen some Russian coaches have a short talk session with a weightlifter and then see the weightlifter lift more weight than he could before the session. This is a sharp distinction from what one typically encounters in the US where the most effective work is in the areas of relaxation, eliminating the "yip's" and reducing anxiety.

A few words must be said about the mental aspects of sports. All too often we hear various athletes and teams talk about the emotional component. It is not uncommon to hear them say that the game is 90% mental and 10% physical.

This is erroneous. The physical plays a very important role in regard to the emotional. For novice athletes and even for up and coming athletes, developing ones physical abilities and skills to a higher level automatically ensures greater confidence which then allows the athlete to perform on a higher level. Skill development and confidence in your skills, i.e. knowing that you can do what you must do when needed is a very important component of the psychological aspects of play.

This is where I believe many professional teams miss out on the training. It becomes obvious if you closely examine the comments made by losing pitchers and other players after a loss. For example, it is common to read that a pitcher "lost his command" or" lost his control" or "left the pitch up high" or that his curveball was not working or some other similar happenstance. These comments indicate that the pitcher did not have the ability to reproduce the same pitch over and over. This is why all teams, if they wanted to prevent this, need to do visual biomechanical analyses to determine what changes had taken place in their technique. The same would apply to other players in regard to their hitting, throwing or running.

If teams were to do this and the players became more consistent in being able to execute optimal performance on a regular basis, the teams would be much more successful. It should also be obvious that if players were able to increase the reliability of their skills, their confidence levels would be extremely high and there probably wouldn't be any need for working on the mental aspects. Most of these would be taken care of automatically as the player is able to perform more reliably which automatically creates more self confidence.

However, there are still instances when the skills and confidence levels are already developed to a high level, that the psychological or mental aspects of game play become very important especially in major completion such as the

Olympics. The number of athletes who are on this level however, is fairly low. The main point here is that you should not think that mental aspects are more important than the physical, they are not. You must perfect the physical before you can have the most effective mental. If you work on the mental aspects without having the commensurate physical abilities and skills, the mental training will be of little value.

Other examples and a broader view of Russian psychological training can be found in a compilation of Russian articles soon to be published. Contact Dr. Yessis at dryessis@dryessis.com for more information on availability.

A sampling of titles include:

Developing Specialized Perceptions

Developing mental motor images

Teaching methods of controlling negative emotional states

Objective and subjective factors in preparing an athlete for a specific competition

Self regulation of negative internal states

Emotion and other psychological factors

Psychological preparation of wrestlers

Operative psychological aid to a hockey player

Ways of regulating a teams psychological state

Developing volitional qualities, correcting negative character traits

Autogenic training and autosuggestions before competition

An operative method of assessing athletes' psychological states

Chapter 8:
Nutritional Guidelines for Improving Performance

You are what you eat." It's a popular cliche, but in the world of sports, it may be particularly true. As important as a proper physical and psychological training program is for the athlete, his or her nutrition can be an equally critical element in determining whether and when peak performance is achieved.

If you take sports seriously, you are probably not nutritionally ignorant. You may be quite conscientious about what you eat, relying mainly on healthy, balanced meals from the major food groups. And it has probably made a positive difference in your competitive level.

But you may not be doing all that you can to turn nutrition into an ally in your athletic endeavors. While helping American athletes analyze their own diets, I've found that even during serious training periods, too many athletes have moments of carelessness. Pressured by time or tempted by chocolate sundaes, they may deviate from the food choices they know are best for them.

Unfortunately, any negative impact that your diet may now be having will not be noticeable immediately. You may feel you're just fine on your present diet, without any indication that even slight alterations in what and when you eat might give you the additional edge you've been seeking.

So what dietary changes should you be thinking about? As in many other areas already described in this book, the Soviets are far ahead of us in answering this question, thanks to their increased understanding of where a nutritional advantage may come from and how to implement it. The U.S. has carried out many fine studies concerning the nutritional needs of the average person, but comparatively little dealing with athletes, particularly the elite ones. Scientists in the U.S.S.R. have done a far superior job of investigating the role of caloric intake, vitamins, minerals, trace elements, protein, fat, and carbohydrates in athletic performance.

Soviet studies have shown that, with a maximal diet, energy increases, resulting in a greater work capacity and improved recuperation time; and that fatigue is more effectively managed because the body has more foodstuffs to utilize to get back to the homeostatic state.

In many cases, Soviet researchers have broken down their nutritional data for individual sports and particular competitive situations. It has become a sophisticated science, so that if you truly are what you eat, then it's not surprising that the Soviets so often outperform their competitors from the West.

FILLING YOUR NUTRITIONAL NEEDS

First of all, your energy needs (and thus your food intake) will vary, depending on your sport. If endurance events, such as long-distance running, are your specialty, Soviet studies show that your training regimen will probably result in an expenditure of up to 5,000-6,000 kilocalories per day. That's two to two and a half times the energy you'd consume if you didn't participate in sports. Volleyball players expend 4,500-5,500 kcal per day, water poloists use up about 3,800 kcal, and cyclists (depending on distances covered) utilize between 4,380 and 9,000 kcal.

Ideally, you should maintain an energy *balance* each day. That means that your daily energy expenditure should roughly match your energy intake. You can judge rather simply whether your own diet is adequate in calories; if you're losing weight while on a rigorous workout schedule, you are probably not consuming enough calories.

To complicate matters a bit, recent Soviet studies seem to indicate that during the preparatory periods of training, it's wise periodically to decrease the caloric intake by 10 to 15 percent, while leaving the energy expenditure as before. By doing this, food will be better absorbed and digested, and training effectiveness will rise. Try this for seven to ten days, and if it appears to benefit you, repeat it at frequent intervals as you train.

But there's obviously more to a good diet than caloric intake. Sufficient levels of proteins, fats, and carbohydrates are essential, and if there's a deficiency or an imbalance in any of them, your performance—and ultimately your health—can suffer.

Take protein, for instance. Soviet studies clearly show that proteins do not have a major impact upon energy levels. But if an athlete's daily diet does not include enough protein, muscle activity will be adversely affected, and the process of biochemical restitution will be retarded. In short, protein is essential for muscle recovery and growth, and especially important if you're seeking to improve your strength.

For athletes, the closer the food protein is to the protein composition of human muscle, the greater its value. Up to 95 percent of meat protein, for example, is assimilated by the body, compared to 85 to 90 percent of the protein in eggs and milk, and 65 to 80 percent of the protein in most kinds of fish.

But as important as animal protein—particularly meat products—may be, vegetable sources should not be ignored. True, most athletes give preference to meat, fish, and cottage cheese at the expense of vegetables, potatoes, and bread. Yet most research in the U.S.S.R. indicates that the day's meals should be composed of approximately equal portions of animal and vegetable protein, in order to stimulate tissue building and increase muscle strength in training. Keep in mind that vegetable protein differs from animal protein in its amino acid structure—and the body needs both.

To facilitate the assimilation and synthesis of protein in the body, a sufficient quantity of carbohydrates must be consumed as well. Thus, almost immediately after a long and rigorous workout, during which large amounts of protein are typically lost, you should consume adequate amounts of fluids, mineral salts, and carbohydrates. Then about an hour later, you should eat foods rich in protein, while continuing to consume a sizable amount of carbohydrates in the next four to six hours. This will ensure a rapid restoration before the next workout.

Carbohydrates are the basic source of energy that permits muscles to remain active. In fact, certain tissues such as nerves can obtain their energy only from carbohydrates.

Like carbohydrates, fats also supply the body with energy. They are also higher in caloric content than the other food categories (supplying about three to four times the calories of carbohydrates and proteins). As fats break down, they are a potent source of energy.

Butter is often recommended for Soviet athletes because it is the most easily assimilated fat. Vegetable oil in amounts of 20 to 25 grams (0.7 to 0.87 ounces) per day is also considered essential, since it contains unsaturated fatty acids that are needed for proper utilization of the body's own fats and for the functioning of the brain cells. Salads with vegetable oil and fish canned in oil are also frequently suggested for athletes.

To maintain a balanced diet, you should aim toward a proper ratio of the main classes of nutrients. While proteins, fats, and carbohydrates are often suggested in a ratio of 1:1:4 in the U.S., the Soviets have discovered that the ideal ratios can vary considerably from one sport to the next.

An athlete's daily nutritional requirements can also vary depending on the intensity of his or her training. When the workouts are of low intensity, the Soviets have found that 1.4 to 2.0 grams (0.05 to 0.07 ounces) of protein per kilogram of body mass per day is sufficient. But during intensive training periods, a greater amount of protein is required (2.2 to 2.9 grams — 0.08 to 0.1 ounces — per kilogram of body mass). Animal protein should comprise no less than 55 to 65 percent of the total amount of protein consumed. (See Table 9.)

TABLE 9 Daily energy requirements of athletes and main food substances in periods of heavy and intense training (per kg of body mass)

Kind of Sports	Protein, g	Fat, g	Carbohy-drates, g	Caloric Value, Cal
Gymnastics, figure skating	2.2–2.5	1.7–1.9	8.6–9.75	59–66
Track and field:				
Sprints, jumps	2.3–2.5	1.8–2.0	9.0–9.8	62–67
Middle- and long-distance running	2.4–2.8	2.0–2.1	10.3–12	69–78
Super-long-distance running and sports walking for 20–50km	2.5–2.9	2.0–2.2	11.2–13	73–84
Swimming and water polo	2.3–2.5	2.2–2.4	9.5–10.0	67–72
Weightlifting, throwing	2.5–2.9	1.8–2.0	10.0–11.8	66–77
Wrestling and boxing	2.4–2.8	1.8–2.2	9.0–11.0	62–75
Rowing (academic, canoe, kayak)	2.5–2.7	2.0–2.3	10.5–11.3	70–77
Soccer, hockey	2.4–2.6	2.0–2.2	9.6–10.4	66–72
Basketball, volleyball	2.3–2.4	1.8–2.0	9.5–10.8	63–71
Cycling:				
Track (velo-drome)	2.3–2.5	1.8–2.0	10.8–11.8	69–75
Road racing	2.5–2.7	2.0–2.1	12.2–14.3	77–87
Equestrianism	2.1–2.3	1.7–1.9	8.9–10.0	60–66
Sailing	2.2–2.4	2.1–2.2	8.5–9.7	62–68
Shooting	2.2–2.4	2.0–2.1	8.3–9.5	60–67
Skiing:				
Downhill	2.3–2.5	1.9–2.2	10.2–11.0	67–74
Cross-country	2.4–2.6	2.0–2.4	11.5–12.6	74–82
Speed skating	2.5–2.7	2.0–2.3	10.0–10.9	69–74

During the days of actual competition, it's extremely important that the food you consume is of the highest quality. The Soviets suggest not only adequate calories in the diet, but also food that is easily assimilated. They recommend that you supplement your meals those days with honey and milk products. Chicken is a particularly good meat choice.

And how close to competition should you eat? A lot of this is personal preference, but Soviet nutritionists generally find that the final meal should be consumed two to four hours prior to the start of competition.

During an endurance event such as a marathon or speed walking, you should be concerned mainly with replenishing your fluid reserves. To fight dehydration, the Soviets have their athletes take 400 to 500 ml (14 to 17 ounces) of fluids about twenty-five to thirty minutes before the start of the race. During the event itself, the ideal fluid consumption level seems to be about 100 to 200 ml (3.5 to 7 ounces) of liquid four to six times.

Because of heavy perspiration during a long running event like a marathon, you're not going to be able to replenish everything that's lost by drinking the liquids available along the race route. While fluid losses occur at a rate of 30 to 40 ml (1 to 1.4 ounces) per minute, fluids cannot move through the stomach any faster than 25 ml (0.9 ounces) per minute. However, frequent fluid intake — even when you don't feel thirsty — can still minimize the negative impact of perspiration on your work capacity and decrease the chances of physiological complications.

While the actual content of the fluid you drink depends largely on personal preference, the Soviets recommend adding sugar or honey to the water, juice, or tea that is being consumed. Some athletes also add lemon juice, mineral salts, and various vitamin mixtures (including ascorbic acid) to their drinks.

MAKING THE MOST OF SUPPLEMENTS

The typical American coach will tell you that his athlete doesn't need additional vitamins and minerals. If you read the professional sports journals in this country, you'll find that he's simply following the advice of our own nutritional experts.

But the Soviets disagree, and they have the research to back them up. Their data show that the high-level athlete's diet—even if it is balanced—usually cannot supply him or her with all the vitamins and minerals used up in heavy training or competition. One recent Soviet study showed that while training for endurance events, athletes typically experienced a deficiency in *all* vitamins except vitamin A. Therefore behind the Iron Curtain, particularly during periods of heavy workouts, supplements are as much a part of the training table as any other nutrient.

In the West, there is no real consensus about the daily requirements of vitamins and minerals even for average individuals, much less athletes. But in the U.S.S.R., using data from sophisticated research, computers are determining precisely how much vitamin A, vitamin C, iron, and calcium each athlete needs, depending on his or her sport (see Tables 10 and 11).

TABLE 10 Daily Requirement of Vitamins for Athletes

Sport	Ascorbic acid (C), mg	Thiamine (B_1), mg	Ribofla-vin (B_2), mg	Panto-thenic acid (B_5), mg	Pyri-doxine (B_6), mg	Folacin (B_9), mkg	Cyanocoba-lamin (B_{12}), mkg	Nicotinic Acid (B_3), mg	A, mg	E, mg
Gymnastics, Figure skating	120–175	2.5–3.5	3.0–4.0	16	5–7	400–500	0.003–0.006	21–35	2.0–3.0	15–30
Track and field:										
Sprints, jumps	150–200	2.8–3.6	3.6–4.2	18	5–8	400–500	0.004–0.008	30–36	2.5–3.5	22–26
Middle- and long-distance runs	180–250	3.0–4.0	3.6–4.8	17	6–9	500–600	0.005–0.01	32–42	3.0–3.8	25–40
Super-long runs, sports walking, 20–50km	200–35-	3.2–5.0	3.5–5.0	19	7–10	500–600	0.006–0.01	32–45	3.2–3.8	28–45
Swimming and water polo	150–250	2.9–3.9	3.4–4.5	18	6–8	400–500	0.004–0.008	25–40	3.0–3.8	28–40
Weightlifting, throwing	175–210	2.5–4.0	4.0–5.5	20	7–10	450–600	0.004–0.009	25–45	2.8–3.8	20–35
Wrestling and boxing	175–250	2.4–4.0	3.8–5.2	20	6–10	450–600	0.004–0.009	25–45	3.0–3.8	20–30

TABLE 10 Daily Requirement of Vitamins for Athletes (*continued*)

Sport	Ascorbic acid (C), mg	Thiamine (B₁), mg	Riboflavin (B₂), mg	Pantothenic acid (B₅), mg	Pyridoxine (B₆), mg	Folacin (B₉), mkg	Cyanocobalamin (B₁₂), mkg	Nicotinic Acid (B₃), mg	A, mg	E, mg
Rowing (academic, canoe, kayak)	200–300	3.1–4.5	3.6–5.3	19	5–8	500–600	0.005–0.01	30–45	3.0–3.8	25–45
Soccer and hockey	180–220	3.0–3.9	3.9–4.4	18	5–8	400–500	0.004–0.008	30–35	3.0–3.6	25–30
Basketball and volleyball	190–240	3.0–4.2	3.8–4.8	18	6–9	450–550	0.005–0.008	30–40	3.2–3.7	25–35
Cycling: Track (velodrome)	150–250	3.5–4.0	4.0–4.6	17	6–7	400–500	0.005–0.01	23–40	2.8–3.6	28–35
Road racing	200–350	4.0–4.8	4.6–5.2	19	7–10	500–600	0.005–0.01	32–45	3.0–3.8	30–45
Equestrianism	130–175	2.7–3.0	3.0–3.5	15	5–7	400–450	0.003–0.006	24–30	2.0–2.7	20–30
Sailing	150–200	3.1–3.6	3.6–4.2	15	5–8	400–450	0.002–0.006	30–35	2.8–3.7	20–30
Shooting	130–180	2.6–3.5	3.0–4.0	15	5–7	400–450	0.002–0.006	25–35	3.5–4.0	20–30
Skiing: Downhill	150–210	3.4–4.4	3.8–4.6	18	7–9	450–500	0.005–0.008	30–40	3.0–3.6	20–40
Cross-country	200–350	3.8–4.9	4.3–5.6	19	6–9	500–600	0.006–0.01	34–45	3.0–3.8	30–45
Speed skating	150–200	3.4–3.9	3.8–4.4	18	7–9	400–550	0.004–0.01	30–40	2.5–3.5	20–40

TABLE 11 Daily need of athletes for some mineral substances (mg)

Sport	Calcium	Phosphorus	Iron	Magnesium	Potassium
Gymnastics, figure skating	1,000–1,400	1,250–1,750	25–35	400–700	4,000–5,000
Track and field:					
Sprints, jumps	1,200–2,100	1,500–2,500	25–40	500–700	4,500–5,500
Middle- and long-distance runs	1,600–2,300	2,000–2,800	30–40	600–800	5,000–6,500
Super-long distance runs, sport walking, 20 and 50km	1,800–2,800	2,200–3,500	35–45	600–800	5,500–7,000
Swimming, water polo	1,200–2,100	1,500–2,600	25–40	500–700	4,500–5,500
Weightlifting, throwing	2,000–2,400	2,500–3,000	20–35	500–700	4,000–6,500
Wrestling, boxing	2,000–4,000	2,500–3,000	20–38	500–700	5,000–6,000
Rowing (academic, canoe, kayak)	1,800–2,500	2,500–3,000	20–38	600–800	5,000–6,500
Soccer, hockey	1,200–1,800	1,500–2,250	25–30	450–650	4,500–5,500
Basketball, volleyball	1,200–1,900	1,500–2,370	25–40	450–650	4,000–6,000
Cycling: Track (velodrome)	1,300–2,300	1,600–1,800	25–30	500–700	4,500–6,000
Road racing	1,800–2,700	2,250–3,400	30–40	600–800	5,000–7,000
Equestrianism	1,000–1,400	1,250–1,750	25–30	400–800	4,000–5,000
Sailing	1,200–2,200	1,500–2,750	20–30	400–700	4,500–5,500
Shooting	1,000–1,400	1,250–1,750	20–30	400–500	4,000–5,000
Skiing: Downhill	1,200–2,300	1,500–2,800	25–60	500–700	4,500–5,500
Cross-country	1,800–2,600	2,300–3,250	30–48	600–800	5,000–7,000
Speed skating	1,200–2,300	1,500–2,800	25–40	500–700	4,500–6,500

234

Here is a brief rundown on the most important athletic-related vitamin supplements, and the role they play in your own body:

* Vitamin A can improve the condition of your skin and mucous membranes, and promote healing of minor injuries.

* Vitamin BI (thiamine), by assisting in the utilization of carbohydrates in the tissue, aids in the recovery process from muscle and nerve fatigue. It can also increase your capacity for heavy physical activity.

* Vitamin B_2 (riboflavin) can help you withstand the burdens of stress and can minimize your chances of developing allergies.

* Vitamin C (ascorbic acid) keeps the body toned up, and as it assists in tissue metabolism, it can help speed up regenerative processes after training and competition,

* Vitamin D aids in the building and strengthening of bone tissue and in accelerating regenerative processes.

* Vitamin E helps increase the elasticity of muscular tissue and thus minimizes the risk of injury.

Minerals should not be overlooked either, although at least in the U.S., they certainly have not received the emphasis and publicity that vitamins have. Without increasing a range of minerals in your body and bloodstream, your capacity for physical work will not rise.

If you have a vitamin or mineral deficiency, you'll first notice it from your inability to recover rapidly after competition. Next, you'll see some decline in your work capacity, and finally, illnesses may develop.

In planning your own vitamin and mineral supplements, keep in mind that particularly heavy training periods, your intake of these additional nu should increase as much as twofold. The more work you do, the greate , ___ need for vitamins.

Mineral salts are another supplement that may be important for proper and rapid restoration. True, Western researchers believe that additional salts are totally unnecessary, even for ultramarathon runners, and are even contraindicated since they may increase blood viscosity and blood pressure, as well as contribute to dehydration. They point to studies in the 1950s and 1960s conducted in South African mines where workers labored in 90-degree temperatures and high humidity.

However, a growing body of Soviet research thinks otherwise. It suggests that mineral salts can be helpful while running marathons (as mentioned earlier), and at other times as well. These salts seem to stimulate normal biochemical reactions within the body, as well as assist in muscle contractability and other bodily processes. To keep mineral salt levels at an optimum level, especially during hot weather and during lengthy training sessions, many Soviet coaches are now recommending the use of two to three supplementary salt tablets.

Soviet sports nutritionists have also developed several innovative drinks — ranging from albumen carbohydrate to electrolyte potions — that contain many kinds of trace elements and have proven quite effective for their athletes. These supplements, as well as refreshing the athlete, help both the preparation and restoration processes.

Some of these liquid dietary supplements are easy to make at home. Here are the ingredients of one that is particularly popular in the U.S.S.R.:

* 50 grams (1.8 ounces) of sugar
* 50 grams (1.8 ounces) of glucose
* 40 grams (1.4 ounces) of fruit juice or berry juice
* 0.5 gram (.02 ounce) of aspartic acid (a plant-source amino acid)
* 2 grams (.07 ounce) of acid phosphate of sodium
* 1 gram (.04 ounce) of salt
* 200 ml (7 ounces) of water

The Soviets recommend that this drink be taken one to two hours before competition, in the intervals between performances, and during the recovery period.

The following drink is most effective immediately after the end of an event:

* Dissolve 100 grams (3.5 ounces) of sugar in an 8-ounce glass of water;
* Add ten drops of a pharmaceutical preparation of hydrochloric acid to the solution to provide a pleasant sourish taste (and to speed up gastric-juice secretion slowed down by muscular work);
* Boil the mixture for twenty minutes, which results in a blend of glucose and fructose; and
* Add 0.5 gram (.02 ounce) of vitamin C and up to 8 grams (.3 ounce) of citric acid.

Some of the other Soviet mixtures are more complex, but are worth the effort. For instance, the following drink should be taken thirty to sixty minutes before an intense training session:

*   120 grams (4.2 ounces) of sour cream, 60 grams (2.1 ounces) of sunflower-seed oil, and 1 egg yolk, mixed;

*   100 grams (3.5 ounces) of orange juice, 25 grams (.9 ounce) of cherry preserves, and 50 grams (1.8 ounces) of lemon juice, added to the mixture and beaten well. Enjoy!

Soviet athletes also often turn to a carbohydrate-mineral drink called the "Olympia," which is commercially available in the U.S.S.R., and is used to replenish lost mineral salts. The ingredients below are prepared in boiling water and cooled before consumption:

* Granulated sugar 285 g (9.9 ounces)
* Glucose 500 g (18 ounces)
* Black currant jam 170.7 g (6 ounces)
* Citric acid 14.75 g (.5 ounce)
* Sodium chloride 2.5 g (.1 ounce)
* Potassium phosphate 3.5 g (.1 ounce)
* Magnesium chloride 4.25 g (.2 ounce)
* Sodium glutamate 5 g (.2 ounce)
* Calcium glycerophosphate 4.3 g (.2 ounce)
* Ascorbic acid 2.5 g (.1 ounce)

On a day-to-day basis, try to include about 2 to 2.5 liters (2.5 to 3 quarts) of water in your diet. That includes the water in tea, milk, and soups, and the water contained in fruits, vegetables, and various dishes.

FINE-TUNING YOUR NUTRITIONAL PROGRAM

Not everyone needs the same dietary program. You have to learn to adjust your diet, based on the needs of your own sport and the rigors of your training and competitive schedule.

By paying attention to body feedback—particularly to symptoms such as fatigue—you'll get a good sense of whether your nutritional program is up to par. Common sense is also a great aid: moderation in anything you eat is a good idea. Also, some athletes simply need more calories than others, depending on their sport; jumpers, for instance, require perhaps half the calories runners do. The appropriate caloric intake is important, since extra calories equal extra weight.

Table 12 shows the types of guidelines that athletes in the U.S.S.R. are routinely asked to follow. Based on studies, it provides daily portions of various food products for top-level track athletes training for endurance events. The chart is prepared for women weighing 130 pounds and men weighing 158 pounds. If you weigh less or more, make corresponding corrections before applying it to your own nutritional program. The more you weigh, the more calories you need to maintain that weight.

The Soviets are getting away from the widely held American belief that to gain strength, you need to eat much more than normal, which will bulk you up and prepare you for rigorous training. Nutritionists in the U.S.S.R. have learned that when a regimen like this is followed for an extended period of time, athletes tend to develop excessive fat. So they eat a balanced diet with proper supplements instead, and are able to meet their training goals while ending up slimmer and trimmer.

**TABLE 12 Basic food products in the daily ration of
runners training for endurance events**

| Food | Wt of products, grams | |
	Women	Men
Lean meat	250–300	300–400
Fish	50–75	75–100
Eggs	50	50
Butter	40–50	50–60
Milk, sour cream	400–600	500–700
Cheese, 30% fat	30–50	50–75
Cottage cheese, nonfat	75–100	100–125
Potatoes	200–250	250–300
Fresh vegetables	300–350	350–400
Fresh fruits	200–250	250–300
Fruit juices	500–600	600–700
Bread and flour products	400–450	450–500
Sweets and honey	120–150	150–180
Mineral water	600–800	800–1,000

As a general rule, the Soviets have also discovered that the most useful eating pattern involves four meals a day. This approach permits the best assimilation and digestion of your food. About 20 to 25 percent of the day's ration are eaten during the early morning meal, 15 to 20 percent are consumed at the second breakfast, 30 to 35 percent during the midday meal, and 20 to 25 percent in the evening meal. Don't allow more than four to five hours to pass between each of the day's meals, and no more than twelve hours between the evening meal and breakfast.

Don't eat immediately before a training session, since a full stomach raises the diaphragm, forcing the cardiovascular and respiratory systems to work harder. Avoid eating just after training, too. Few gastric juices are secreted during this time, so you should wait twenty to thirty minutes for normal digestive conditions to reappear.

One final point: weather and training conditions can also affect nutritional programs. If you're an endurance runner, hot weather means less fat and carbohydrate and a corresponding drop in caloric intake. At the same time, increase the amount of proteins and vitamins you consume. About 70 to 100 grams (2.5 to 3.5 ounces) of fluids should be drunk in small swallows every twenty to thirty minutes during training.

By contrast, in cold weather, there is greater heat loss, and thus the endurance runner in particular should be aiming toward an increase in energy potential. Therefore, food volume should rise, with an increase in all nutritional components, especially carbohydrates and vitamins.

If you're training at high altitudes, your main concern is insufficient oxygen in the air, which you feel most strongly during the first seven to ten days as you become acclimatized. In this situation, the Soviets suggest that you significantly decrease the amount of fats in your diet, while increasing carbohydrates. This makes sense since obtaining energy from fats utilizes much more oxygen than energy from carbohydrates. Also, increase the levels of proteins and vitamin B food products (lean meat, cottage cheese, liver, coarse-ground bread) in your diet.

By adhering to recommendations like these, nutrition will become an important ally in your athletic life.

Chapter 8 Addendum

There have been many advances in nutrition in the past 21 years, with many taking place in the U.S. However, most of the findings and research has not dealt specifically with athletes but with the general population. Some of the information has implications for athletes, but the basic tenets of nutrition for athletes as brought out in the original text still hold true today. Nutrition plays a very important role in recovery, for producing energy for performance, for replacing what was used up in the work, in the healing and treatment of injuries, and damage to the tissues etc.

One of the more important findings has been on the effects of using natural whole food vitamin and mineral supplements as opposed to their synthetic versions. However, the conclusion that whole food supplements are much more effective (and even have different effects!), still has not permeated mainstream thinking or gotten to most athletes. Because of this, I strongly recommend that you closely examine the supplements you use and avoid those that are not made out of whole foods. Simply read the label and if you read names of different foods from which it is composed, then you know that it is made out of whole foods. If instead you see many chemical names then you know that it is synthetic.

According to various nutrition specialists, balanced diets are back in for all athletes. It has been found that overemphasizing any one group of nutrients as for example, using high carbohydrate diets are not as beneficial as once believed. When athletes carbohydrate load or use a diet heavy in carbohydrates, they teach the body to rely on carbohydrates for energy. However, carbohydrates are burned up very quickly and if you run a long race or must play a very long game with overtimes, you typically will not have enough high level energy to finish the competition well. But, if athletes had a balanced diet and trained their body to rely more on fats, which produce twice the amount of energy, it would enable them to complete the race or game without "running out of gas".

What confuses the issue are the many recommendations given by sports nutrition companies. They often do research to promote the value of their own products rather than helping to clear up confusion in the field, especially in regard to products for energy and recovery. As a result, there are many claims for products that supposedly give you more energy (even if it is only for a short period as for example, caffeine) or help you recover faster as for example, carbohydrate and protein mixtures. There's no question that many of these products do as they say, but whether they help you over long periods of time as in a marathon or even over a period of a year or two is left unanswered.

In addition, Russian as well as American nutritionists found that natural sea salt that contains a balance of most minerals that the body needs, is very effective in replacing the minerals that the body needs after hard or long workouts. This is especially important for athletes who must perform in the heat or for extended periods of time and who perspire considerably. By taking a pinch of pure sea salt the athlete is able to continue performing at a high level for extended periods or to recover more quickly after a hard workout.

A key nutritional factor to be emphasized here is to use, as much as possible, whole, organic foods. With sorrow, too much of today's food supply is not grown this way and thus often lacks important nutrients. In addition, commercially grown foods often have chemical residue, may be bio engineered (the full effects of which may not be known for many years) or are irradiated to provide longer shelf life. Irradiation however, kills the food. For example, plant an organic potato and it will grow; one that has been irradiated, will not! Does this not constitute a dead vegetable? This is why the Russians and to a good extent, Europe has been very reluctant to embrace these new technologies.

Many products such as fruits do not have the nutrients that they should because they are picked too early in order to have a longer shelf life. This is not even taking into consideration the lack of taste that most early picked fruits have. In addition, there has been an increasing number of recalls or problems arising with the handling of food. This is appearing to be a major problem not only in the processing plants but also in restaurants.

Thus, as much as possible, it is recommended that your nutrition be based on sources where you know the food will be good, or as good as one could expect, rather than taking chances on getting stomach or some other digestive problems when training. Keep in mind that it is now common to find many athletes who experience food poisoning, abdominal pain, nausea or vomiting, etc. and cannot perform or do not perform as well as hoped for in major competition.

The conclusion is that you should seek out nutritionists or medical professionals who specialize in the use of nutrients for energy and recovery to enhance your workouts and/or playing, healing and treatment of injuries. Many whole food supplements are very effective in these areas. This is extremely important for athletes in order to maintain high level intense training regimes, to prepare for competition and to compete. For more information on the use of nutrients in recovery as recommended by the Russians read Sports Restoration and Massage.

An area in which the Russians did extensive research was in adaptogens, natural plant products that help the body protect itself against various stressors. They also help the body to adapt to high stress. Multiple plant products have been found to be especially valuable and include many herbs. They are used extensively by Russian athletes to help offset fatigue and maintain better focus and concentration. The adaptogens are especially valuable when athletes must travel long distances for competition as they help to reduce travel stress and jet lag. In addition, the adaptogens are often used to prepare athletes for a great amount of work during high volume or high intensity training cycles.

Some researchers have found that combined adaptogens do not have any side effects and can help restore weakened functions of the body. This in turn creates conditions for realizing the optimal work capacity of an athlete. However, the Russians are also the first to tell you that the adaptogens work mainly in carefully planned individualized programs. They believe that it is not always desirable to use adaptogens or other restorative measures on a regular basis because they may impair the body's ability to adapt efficiently on its own. Consequently, they recommend that partial restoration is essential at different times and for different reasons. They also stress that adaptogens have different effects when taken at different times of the day, after different training loads, at different climatic stages and so on.

Adaptogens are not unique to Russia and can now be found in many different countries including the US. Some of the more common ones include Eleutherococcus, schizandra, pantocrine, elton, leveton, tincture of Chinese lemon tree, velvet antler, saparal, mumie, extract of rose root stone crop, adaptozol and tonedrin. There are also whole food supplements that act as excellent adaptogens. Most state-of-the-art nutritionists should be able to guide you in this area. It is too complex to fully report on in this text.

Chapter 9:

MAKING THE MOST OF SOVIET RESTORATIVE MEASURES

After a particularly rigorous workout, do you sometimes feel as though you'll never be able to muster the energy for the following day's session? Or during the competitive season, do you find yourself so fatigued in the final weeks that you seem unable to perform up to your capabilities?

This is a common phenomenon among athletes, particularly those who haven't learned effective techniques for recuperation. And in an era when training regimens are becoming so intense and athletes are so often performing at record-breaking levels, the process of recovery and restoration can't be overlooked.

Even a decade ago, the marathon was thought to be the ultimate endurance event, and the training it required placed enormous demands on athletes. Today the triathlon has emerged as an even greater challenge. The Iron Man triathlon includes not only a marathon, but also 2.4 miles of swimming and 120 miles of cycling. For most of us, just thinking about it is exhausting.

As the athletes of today train and compete longer and harder than ever, they must learn to use recuperative techniques so their bodies can withstand and cope with the increased "loads." As one Soviet sports researcher has written, "Further increases in physical loads (as is continually happening) lead to such changes in the athlete that they go beyond physiological norms, worsen the functional state and lower work ability. . . . Because of this . . . the most effective means for raising the work ability of the athlete is wide use of various methods of restoration."

Studies in the U.S.S.R. show that recovery techniques actually work on three different levels. First of all, there is some recuperation that goes on during the workout or the competition itself. Then recovery begins in earnest immediately after the workout ends, with the excretion of waste products and the replacement of expended resources.

Finally, there is a delayed recovery, which optimally could raise the athlete to competitive levels higher than he or she has ever achieved before. Soviet research in physiology and endocrinology shows that during this so-called "super compensation" phase, the body deposits *extra* energy stores in addition to those lost during exercise. This process makes growth in the capability of the athlete possible—allowing him or her to run faster, jump higher, or lift more weight.

Restoration techniques have become so sophisticated behind the Iron Curtain that Soviet athletes now utilize special equipment built just for this purpose. Electrostimulators, for instance, are used routinely to massage the muscles electrically. Electrodes are placed on the muscles and a current is transmitted through them, causing them to contract. Much more precisely than in the U.S., the intensity and the duration of the current can be adjusted, along with variations in amplitude and frequency, achieving a variety of effects—from improving local blood circulation and metabolic processes to reducing fatigue and increasing muscle strength.

The Soviets also make wide use of ultrasound machines for restoration. These devices enable microtraumas that a trainer or physician might not even notice to heal more rapidly. (These microtraumas are believed to occur almost routinely in extremely hard workouts.) Also, because of ultrasound's analgesic properties, pain in the tendons and ligaments is decreased or eliminated.

There are also various types of pressure chambers in wide use in the U.S.S.R. By altering atmospheric pressure within the chamber, these devices can revitalize fatigued or injured parts of the body. An arm or a leg, for instance, might be inserted into the elongated tube of the Kravchenko pressure chamber, after which the external pressure around that limb is reduced. In the process, this local decompression alters blood circulation, tissue respiration, and temperature in a positive way.

That isn't all, however. A separate device permits the entire body to be placed in a much larger chamber, where the athlete can breathe in oxygen under pressure. A study found that when this device was utilized consistently, the work capacity of Soviet swimmers increased 25 percent.

These devices are generally not available in the U.S. for use by athletes. But there are plenty of other restorative approaches available to the American athlete. Many of them are described below, and if you use them consistently, you'll be strides ahead of most of your competitors, who may have never been introduced to them.

MASSAGE

Even the recreational athlete can benefit from Soviet approaches to massage. This is the most widely used restorative measure behind the Iron Curtain, and various forms of it can be utilized. I'm not talking about the leisurely, relaxing type of massage so popular in the U.S. Instead, the Soviets utilize a methodical, scientific system that provides stimulation and therapy for individual needs.

A classical massage given by a well-trained Soviet sports massage practitioner usually takes from forty to fifty minutes. The massage varies depending on the particular sport, with emphasis on different parts of the body. If you're a runner, for instance, most of the attention would be placed on the buttocks and calf muscles; the thighs (especially the posterior surface); the hip, ankle, and knee joints; and the foot. The trunk itself would receive no more than 10 percent of the massage time.

Here are some tips on what Soviet massage practitioners now use on the lower part of the body, which is the focus of attention for runners.

1. Massage of the hip area should begin with stroking and jostling of the muscles. The gluteus muscles should be squeezed and then kneaded. A two-handed grip is usually utilized for circular rubbing with the knuckles, the fists, and the pads of the fingers. The massage of this region is completed with some additional jostling, striking motions, and stroking.

2. The calf muscles should be the focus in working on the legs, using longitudinal movements (short strokes with the pads of the fingers) and nine to twelve consecutive circular motions with the fingers of one hand.

3. Massage of the posterior surface of the thigh should start with two to three stroking motions, followed by vigorous transverse squeezing and then some rubbing (for example, circular and longitudinal motions with the back side of

flexed fingers) Some jostling and stroking movements should then be performed.

4. When moving on to the anterior surface of the thigh, start with two-handed stroking. Squeeze the muscles with both hands.

You do not need an experienced massage practitioner, however, to reap the benefits of a restorative massage. Self-massage, in fact, is almost universally practiced in the U.S.S.R.

Of course, there are some limitations to self-massage. Certain back muscles, for instance, are beyond the reach of your own hands. But research has shown that when used during the warmup before workouts or competition, or about thirty minutes afterward, self-massage can increase the work capacity of the muscles and accelerate their recovery.

In sports that require running and jumping, self-massage is usually limited to the legs. When throwing is also part of the sport, the upper extremities are massaged as well. Try the following techniques as you move from one part of the body to the next:

1. Recline on your side to self-massage the outer thigh. Use straight-line stroking with the fingertips, spiral motions with the base of the palm, and circular rubbing with the cushions of the four fingers.

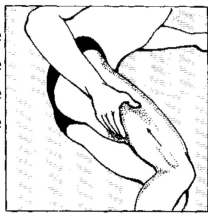

2. Move to a seated position to massage the anterior thigh. The massaged leg should be resting comfortably on the table or couch. Use a variety of circular motions with the thumb pad and the cushions of the four fingers. Also, place the hands on the lower part of the thigh, with one thumb slightly in front of the other. Then squeeze the thumbs back toward the fingers, pressing on the muscles as you do.

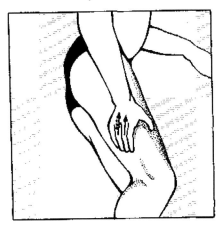

3. Remain in the same position for self-massaging the interior thigh. Use straight-line stroking, and then circular rubbing using the pads of the four fingers and the base of the palms.

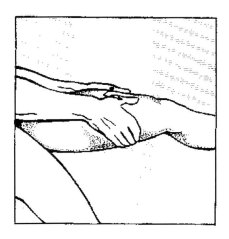 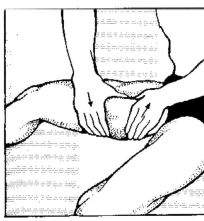

4. Massaging the dorsal surface of the lower leg is performed by grasping the muscle with the thumb on one side and the fingers on the other. Pull the hand away but do not let go, and then perform rotary motions upward.

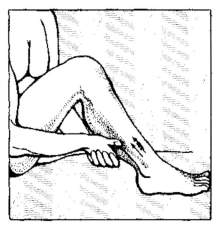

5. To self-massage the buttocks, stand with the massaged leg drawn to the side, with a slight bend at the knee. Your body weight should be placed on the free leg. Using the same-side hand, alternate between some longitudinal stroking and some circular rubbing using the base of the hand and the pads of the four fingers.

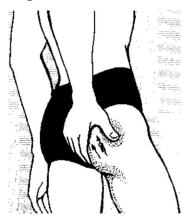

6. The foot can be massaged in a sitting position, with the leg to be worked on bent at the knee, and the other one hanging off the edge of the table or couch. With the palms grasping the foot, and with the thumbs pointing upward, stroke the foot with both hands simultaneously, moving from the tip of the toes toward the heel.

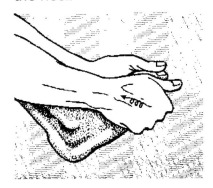

7. To self-massage the shoulders, with the thumb on one side and four fingers on the other, use a circular motion alternating with a pinching maneuver.

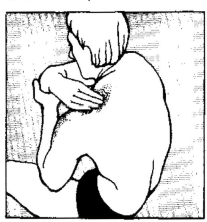

American athletes with whom I have worked find these self-massage techniques enormously helpful. Some have also used vibrational massage, which was developed in the U.S.S.R.; but once again, this requires special equipment. Even so> studies have consistently shown that this "vibromassage" can increase the functional state of the neuromuscular system. If you have access to a sports vibromassager, several minutes with this device (operating at 10 to 15 Hz) can be very effective for restoration. In the Soviet Union, it is used primarily by athletes with big muscle mass (such as weightlifters and wrestlers); other athletes can usually get by with hand massage.

HEAT

The Soviets have perfected the use of saunas, steam baths, and hydrotherapy as part of their restoration programs. But as with massage, these approaches are not intended for leisurely relaxation. They're integral parts of the recuperation process, and the temperature and duration of each session are carefully regulated.

Dry heat in a sauna is the most widely recommended of these approaches. A ten-to-fifteen-minute exposure is usually adequate for recovery of work capacity, although some athletes spend up to twenty minutes after a particularly strenuous training session. The benefits are especially significant for the circulatory and the neuromuscular systems. Muscular pain generated by overtraining often decreases, and saunas also promote rapid removal of wastes from the body.

Based on Soviet studies, here are some guidelines for using saunas as a restorative tool:

* Air temperature in a sauna should not exceed 194 degrees Fahrenheit, with a relative humidity of 5 to 15 percent.
* To maximize its restorative benefits, do not enter the sauna immediately after a workout or competition. It is advisable to wait one to two hours.
* Wash with soap, rinse, and wipe the skin dry before going into the sauna. This will create ideal conditions for the release of sweat and for bodily heat regulation. For the first two to three minutes (of a typical ten minutes) in the

sauna, stay on the lowest benches, and then gradually move to the upper benches. Keep the legs horizontal during most of the time spent at the higher elevations; then sit with the legs lowered in the final two or three minutes before leaving the sauna. After the sauna, consume mineral water or vitaminized drinks to replace the liquids and biological substances that have been lost.

NUTRITION

Given the emphasis on diet and nutrition in the Soviet sports system, it is not surprising that when a restoration program is being created for an athlete, nutrition plays a major role.

One of the most critical components is mineral salts. As mentioned in the previous chapter, it has been found to be particularly important for the normal flow of most biochemical reactions, and for the proper functioning of muscle tissue. Fluids containing mineral salts and glucose (200 to 300 ml, or 7 to 10 ounces) are recommended after a workout of average intensity.

Vitamins have also proved useful for recuperation. In particular, supplementary vitamin C and E are used to aid muscle relaxation, to improve muscle elasticity, and to accelerate the removal of waste from the tissues. Added levels of the B vitamins are recommended for high-altitude workouts, and vitamin E appears useful for athletes who perform speed work. Multivitamin supplements are also suggested during times of the year when workouts are unusually strenuous.

OTHER RESTORATION TECHNIQUES

The Soviets have learned that variety is important to maximize the restoration process. As effective as some of their methods are on their own, combining and alternating different techniques are now commonplace. Table 13 shows how varied and detailed the restoration program is for a weightlifter in a typical weekly training schedule.

There are other approaches in addition to those already described. Acupuncture and acupressure, for instance, are used with increasing frequency, but they require trained practitioners to administer them.

Rest and relaxation techniques are also widely utilized. A Soviet researcher who specializes in studying training and fatigue recently wrote, "The structuring of rest is very important for recovery following fatiguing workloads." When fatigue gradually develops during a lengthy and rigorous training schedule, he considers calm rest and sound sleep essential to allow the body's restorative processes to take place.

The Soviets are also successfully experimenting with hypnotically induced sleep as a restorative device. After a work-out, the athlete enters a tent where a physician places him or her in a hypnotic sleep for two to three minutes. Despite such a short time span, this helps athletes achieve a state of complete rest. As a result, one study shows that swimmers can train between 50 and 100 percent longer, knowing that restoration will occur very quickly after the workout.

Because athletes in the U.S.S.R. recuperate so quickly, thanks to the techniques described in this chapter, they experience a far lower injury rate than their American counterparts. Among athletes who lift a lot of weights (football players, weightlifters, powerlifters), for instance, though injuries to the joints, ligaments, tendons, and muscles occur with alarming frequency to Americans, they are quite rare behind the Iron Curtain.

The Soviets have also found value in several "natural healing" methods of restoration that have been largely scoffed at in the U.S.—from mineral springs to mud baths to (believe it or not) swatting with a collection of birch twigs. I had some personal experience with this during a trip I made to the U.S.S.R. in 1983.

After warming up in a steam bath, I was "treated" to a few swats with birch twigs, which opened up the pores on my back and provided some amazing rejuvenation.

While the "blows" were being administered, my skin stung and turned red as a beet, but afterward I felt wonderfully invigorated.

If you combine a wide variety of recuperative systems, you can enhance your recovery process significantly. Don't be content only with self-massage, for example, as helpful as you may find it. You should also be using saunas, nutrition, and other methods to maximize the benefits in your own training program.

I am always surprised at how little research is being done in the United States in the field of restoration. Though it is an expanding area of study behind the Iron Curtain, some U.S. Olympic sports officials doubt that it has any scientific validity. They don't believe that restorative techniques like those practiced in the Soviet Union can benefit athletes at all.

Whenever I hear that, I suggest that these individuals look at the performances of Soviet athletes in recent years in international competition. I think they speak for themselves.

Chapter 9 Addendum

The information presented in this chapter is as valid today as it was the day it was written. There are however, a few minor additions. For example the marathon is no longer considered the major long-distance event. It is not uncommon to find many runners doing long-distance runs and/or races for 50-100 miles. There are even individuals who run a marathon every day for up to 30 or more days in a row. These are outstanding feats of endurance which require even greater use of restorative measures to help the athlete recover.

Sadly, however, little progress has been made in the area of recovery and restoration in the U.S. For example, the use of oxygenated and pressure chambers to duplicate altitude changes. Most often however, they are used for training purposes, not healing or recovery. There have also been significant advances in various electrical instruments such as more sophisticated electrical stimulation units to treat injuries and enhance healing. The use of saunas and steam baths by athletes may also be increasing although they are still used far less than they should be with many teams.

Most teams still lag behind advances in recovery greatly. The Europeans and Russians are way ahead of us in this area. For example, it is easy to find high tech recovery and rehabilitation centers in many "spas" in Russia and in many European countries. These centers have multiple pools, different types of baths, massage, physical therapy and so on. They are used not only for athletes but also for the general public. Many of these modalities can also be found in specific sports training centers or clubs.

A few words must also be said about Russian massage. It is a hybrid of many successful massage techniques developed in different countries over the years. What is most interesting is that massage originated with the medical profession and considerable research was done on its role in treating different types of patients. Because of the great success had by Soviet doctors, when sports became a major priority, it was understandable that massage would soon be incorporated into the total training of athletes. There were several outstanding individuals such as Birukov, who were pioneers in developing different types of massage for different states of the athlete. As a result, you will be there is now specific massage for relaxing an athlete, for stimulating an athlete, for helping an athlete recover, for preparing an athlete for competition and for treatment of injuries.

For anyone interested in more information and details on the various restorative measures mentioned in the original chapter, I recommend reading *Sports Restoration and Massage* . This book is a compilation of articles translated from the Russian with explanatory and supplementary information presented. It is available from Sports Training, Inc., www.dryessis.com. The book explains in detail how the various restorative/recuperative methods can and should be used not only with athletes in general, but also with athletes in specific sports. It can be of great value to all teams and especially to physical therapists and massage practitioners.

There are 70 articles in *Sports Restoration and Massage* categorized into the following sections:

1. Scientific fundamentals and techniques of restoration
2. Sports massage techniques
3. Specialized massage techniques
4. Electro-therapeutic techniques
5. Barometric restoration techniques
6. Thermal restoration techniques
7. Psychological and sensory restoration techniques
8. Nutritional aspects of restoration

Following are several excerpts to give you an idea of the scope and depth of the articles.

EXCERPTS FROM SPORTS RESTORATION AND MASSAGE

THE SAUNA AS A MEANS OF RESTORATION DURING INTENSE SWIMMING TRAINING

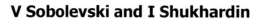

V Sobolevski and I Shukhardin

Plavanye, 15-17, 1980

The sauna appears to be one of the most effective means of restoration in the period of intense training of swimmers. Increased physical work capacity under the influence of a sauna is explained by the positive changes that take place in the highest nerve centres and in the biochemical processes of the muscle contraction. In addition, there is improvement of blood circulation in the peripheral tissues, relaxation of the muscles, activation of the oxygen restorative processes and metabolic reactions, removal (through perspiration) of several end products of the exchange of various substances and toxins and, at the same time, enhanced supply of oxygen and glycogen to the muscles.

In order to make sauna use a quality means of restoration, we conducted a study on highly qualified swimmers in the Neva Swim Centre and in SKIP, in which 35 boys and girls participated. Results of the study showed the favourable effects of using the sauna.

As a result of the study, we can make the following recommendations for using the sauna in different periods of training.

Preparatory Period: During this training period, a large volume of general physical preparation (GPP) is used with a relatively small amount of specialised work in the water. Not infrequently, a feeling of pain is noted in the muscles and there is decreased ability to differentiate muscular effort. When this occurs, the following variant of restoration is recommended: Use the sauna once a week with the temperature at 90 C and relative humidity, 5-15%. The sauna is repeated 2 or 3 times for 10 minutes with a rest interval of 10-15 minutes in between each stay. After each exposure, there is a cool-down shower (water temperature from 20-22 C), alternated with consecutive warm showers for 35 minutes (water temperature 38 C), and local massage.

This variant (III)* is characterised by a small increase in specialised work capacity (endurance), which does not correspond to the main training task in this period. However, use of this variant brings about a steady improvement in general self-feeling of the athletes and increased development of speed-strength qualities.

*Four sauna variants were used: three 10-min exposures, 90 C; Il-two 10-rain exposures, 90 C; Ill-three 10-min exposures, 90 C plus local massage; IV--two 10-rain exposures, 90 C plus general restorative massage.

Competitive Period: In this period, there is an increase in specialised endurance, acquisition of sports form and a significant increase in swimming loads and intensity. Because of this, a 2-3 time exposure for 10 minutes in the sauna with the temperature at 90 C is recommended. The rest period between each exposure is not less than 5 minutes, with moderate cool-down procedures (showers with water temperature from 20-32 C or a shower massage with the water temperature from 36-40 C). This sauna variant (a combination of I and II) is characterized by a significant increase in work capacity. The second variant gives the most favorable results when it is used as a means of rehabilitation.

The Stage immediately before the Main Competitions: For stabilization of sports form at this time, the most effective use of the sauna is variant IV: Air temperature 90 C; relative humidity 5-15%; duration of stay, once or twice for 10 minutes with rest intervals not less than 5 minutes; a quick (30-40 sec) cold shower followed by a warm shower; and general hand massage. For greatest effectiveness, the sauna should be used no later than 15 days prior to competition.

Use of the Sauna in Rehabilitation: The sauna is beneficial when signs of excessive stress and muscle tightness appear during the time when there is a drop in total physical and swimming loads. When used in these conditions, the sauna should have an air temperature of 70 C and relative humidity of 5-15%. The duration of each stay is 10 min, 2 or 3 times. Massage is given after the first and second exposures. A warm shower is then taken for 3-5 mins (water temperature, 36-38 C).

Medical Control When Using the Sauna: The great demands on the functional systems of the swimmer when using the sauna dictate the need for strict medical control and adjustment in the heat load regimes. The most informative and objective criteria for evaluation of the ability to withstand hot sauna conditions is maximum heart rate during the time of perspiration. At this time, it should not go higher than 140 beats/min. Electrocardiography may also be used during the time of being in the sauna or before and after the sauna.

Results of this study and substantiation from studies carried out in other sports allow us to conclude that the alternate use of different variants of hydro- and heat procedures at different stages of training swimmers increases the effectiveness of restorative measures.

Conclusion

We must stress the need for strict observation of the rules for using the sauna, namely:

1. The sauna should only be used by healthy athletes (especially who have no cardiac or respiratory complaints). Use of the sauna as a quality means of rehabilitation and restoration should only be done under medical supervision.

2 . Air temperature in the sauna should not exceed 90 C with a relative humidity of 5-
15%

3. To increase the restorative effect, the athlete should not go into the sauna immediately after execution of physical loads. The best time is 1-2 hours after intense training.

4. Before entering the sauna, it is necessary to wash with soap and to dry fhe skin. This procedure creates the optimal conditions for sweat release and thermal regulation.

5. The stay in the sauna begins on the lowest benches for 2-3 mins, gradually moving higher to the upper benches. On the highest benches, the athlete can either lie down or sit, placing the legs horizontally. During the time of perspiration, it is important to achieve muscular and psychological relaxation. In the last 2 3 mins of being in the hot sauna, it is necessary to sit with lowered legs and only after this, to leave the heat.

6. The sauna stay ends with a 30-40 minute rest, during which time it is necessary to replace the loss of liquids and biologically active substances by using mineral waters and vitaminised drinks. •

DIFFERENTIATED USE OF RESTORATIVE MEASURES FOR WRESTLERS IN THE COMPETITIVE PERIOD

A Birukov, V Savchenko and F Ionov

Teoriya i Praktika Fizicheskoi Kultury, 4:22-23, 1985

In the competitive period it is advisable for wrestlers in devising microcycles of preparation for competition when sports form is maintained or improved, to train on a background of some *non-restoration.* In this case, it is necessary to decrease fatigue only in selected muscle groups and to use methods having a local effect. In restorative microcycles with active rest, one must use complex variants of methods which have general effects on the body. Methods of using the sauna, massage and water procedures should be strictly differentiated. Also, besides the initial functional state and individual essentials of the athlete, the periods and microcycles of preparation should be taken into consideration along with the character of loads. In addition, the phases in which it is necessary to have alternate training sessions with insufficient restoration or supercompensation should be looked at.

Method: The study was carried out during the education-training of the Sambo team in the process of preparation for the Republic team in the VIII Summer Spartakiad of the USSR. There were 22 high level athletes in the study (Master of Sport and Honoured Master of Sport). Each group had 11 men in the experimental and control groups.

The functional state of the wrestlers was controlled with the use of chronax-symmetry, the tapping test, dynamometry of the hand, pulseometry and measurement of arterial pressure. *The coefficient of efficiency of circulation* (CEC) of the blood was calculated as follows:

CEC = (APraax - APmin).HR where APmax is maximum arterial pressure, APmin is minimum arterial pressure and HR is heart rate. The indices studied were taken at the beginning of the educational training camp and at the end of each rnicrocycle. In the experimental group restorative measures were applied according to a method constructed in conjunction with the tasks of the microcycles.

In the process of preparation with relative stabilisation of the volume of training loads, the motor intensity and psychological tension increased in a wavelike fashion, subordinate to the modelled conditions of competitive activity.

In the developmental microcycles after training loads with exclusion of control 'takedowns', fatigue was decreased only in separate muscle groups: the shoulder girdle, arms, back, waist. In the lead-up rnicrocycle the method of acting on the restorative processes was determined in combination with individual indices.

In order to optimise the process of restoration and immediately increasing work capacity, hand or vibrational massage after the first workout was carried out immediately after the end of the session. After the second workout, when it was necessary to increase work capacity on the following day (i.e. in the distant restorative period), restorative massage was used 2-3.5 hours after the loads. In both cases *the principle of alternation of means and methods of massage* was used (specific, general, hand, vibrational, combined).

After peak loads (using controlled take-downs), restoration was applied in three stages:

1. Hand restorative massage (for *5-7* mins) after executing the take-downs
2. Combined and specific massage 2.5-3.5 hours after the loads

3. Sauna and general restorative massage in the morning of the following day, 1.5-2 hours after breakfast.

The method of restorative massage after peak loads follows:

First Stage (5-10 minutes after the training session).

Task: To relax the neuromuscular system and create conditions for optimal restoration.

Methods: Kneading, 10% of the total time of massage, shaking, jostling, 65%, passive movement in the joints with accent on stretching the muscles, 25%.

It should be noted that passive stretching of the muscles can serve as one of the effective methods of increasing work capacity of athletes. Besides the immediate effect, it brings about a cumulative one and also serves to remove muscle pain after intense workouts.

Massage is begun from the spine with light kneading and jostling of the wide, long and trapezius muscles and the hamstrings. The gastrocnemius muscles of both shins are shaken simultaneously, fixing the hands on the feet in the area of the anterior surface of the ankle joints and alternating shaking with passive movement of the knee joints.

The movement is carried out slowly, not sharply, until the sensation of light pain occurs, while paying attention to stretching the muscles of the anterior surface of the thigh. In relation to mobility in the knee joints, they strive to reach the gluteus muscles with the heels of the feet and holding the shins in this position for 3-5 seconds. Further on, passive movement in the ankle joint with emphasis on light stretching of the muscles of the anterior muscles of the shin is carried out.

269

Alternate methods are carried out with the person being massaged lying on his back. The large muscles of the chest are jostled and the arms are shaken alternately, beginning with the entire extremity and afterwards with separate muscles of the upper arm and forearm. *Shaking* is alternated with passive movement of the shoulder, elbow and wrist joints.

After this, with the person being massaged lying on his back, *kneading* and *shaking* is done simultaneously on the anterior and posterior surfaces of the thigh. In this, the closest leg of the person being massaged lies on the thigh of the massage practitioner and the knee stays on the couch.

Jostling is changed with movements in the hip joint. The leg of the perjon being massaged is bent in the knee joint. The hands of the massage practitioner, in fixing the anterior surface of the knee joint, carry out fine oscillating movements, jostling the posterior surface of the thigh and shin.

After this, the wrestler must pick up his leg, extending the knee joint and placing the foot in a position of maximal dorsiflexion. The massage practitioner in fixing the foot in the plantar area lifts the leg of the person being massaged, stretching the muscles of the posterior surface of the thigh and shins, as well as the sciatic nerve.

The massage ends with shaking of the lower extremities. One arm of the massage practitioner fixes the leg of the person being massaged from the side of the Achilles tendon and the other is placed on the foot arch. The massage practitioner pulls the leg toward himself and makes a shaking movement before moving it away and then carrying it back toward himself. While this procedure is being executed, the knee joint should not be flexed.

Second Stage (2-3.5 hours after the control take-downs): In accordance with individual indices specific combined restorative massage is carried out for 20 minutes.

Task: To remove neuromuscular and psychological tension, restore work capacity of separate muscle groups and remove the feeling of pain. Combined massage consists of hand massage and low-frequency vibromassage action with a frequency of 25->15-*25 Hz. Vibromassage is carried out in the area of the neck (portal vein) zone with accent on the

spinal-brain segments of the arm and shoulder girdle. Cervical 3 to thoracic 5 for 7-8 minutes. Vibration is realised with the 'Charodey' apparatus and the frequency of vibration changes from 10 to 100 Hz with changing heat nozzles. Hand massage includes massage of the shoulder girdle, arms, back and waist.

Methods: Combined stroking, 15%; squeezing, 10%; kneading: double circle, double ordinate, with the heels of the palms, 50%; shaking jostling, 25%. Hand massage is done softly at a quiet tempo. Main attention is paid to the regions of muscle and tendon attachment.

Since the arms of the samboist experience great static loads in grabbing the jacket it is necessary to carefully massage the hands and muscles of the forearm, especially the hand flexors.

Third Stage (on the following day 1.5-2 hours after breakfast): sauna and general restorative massage. Temperature of the air in the sauna is maintained within the limits of 90-100 C with the relative humidity at 10-15%. The athletes complete 2-4 stays in the heat for 5 minutes each time. In the breaks between entering the sauna they use contrast showers or baths. General restorative massage is carried out for 20-30 minutes, after the second entry into the sauna. Massage is carried out according to the method previously detailed.

In massage in the sauna it follows to pay especially great attention to the ligamentous system of the joints and the injured parts of the body.

In analysing the data received it is possible to note different dynamics in the physiological indices and in the tempo of their increase in both groups. In the experimental group improvement in the neuromuscular system and heart-circulatory system after the first developmental microcycle was insignificant.

There was a following positive increase in the second microcycle and expression in the lead-up microcycle, which indicates an increased training effect. In the control group the increase of the indices studied from microcycle to microcycle remained the same and insignificant.

Conclusions

1. In the developmental microcycles during the competitive period when sports form is not only maintained but is improving, removing fatigue only in separate muscle groups by considering the effectiveness of restorative measures in close (after the first workout) and later (on the following day) restorative periods, increases the cumulative training effect.

2. One must remember that the term 'restoration[1] does not mean regeneration of all the functions and systems of the body, but restoration of definite more vulnerable functional links which ultimately determine increased physical work capacity.

3. The specific method of restoration described in this article contributed to the successful performance by the Russian samboists in the VII and VIII Summer Spartakiads of the USSR.

EFFECT OF SINUSOIDAL MODULATED CURRENTS ON THE CARDIORESPIRATORY SYSTEM AND WORK CAPACITY

I Dombrovskaya *Kurortologii, Fizioterapii i Lechebnoi Fizicheskoi Kultury,* 5:33-35,1982

It has been noted that physical work capacity of athletes is restored under the influence of massage, hydroelectric baths, decimetre waves and other physical factors (Belaya et al, Zagorskaya, Zhuravleva). The favourable effect of sinusoidal modulated currents (SMC) for cardiovascular diseases is also known. The peripheral circulation of patients is improved, the vessels dilate and blood flow accelerates (Yasnogorodsky, Slepushkina).

This work studies the possibility of using SMC to accelerate the restorative processes in the cardiovascular system in athletes after considerable physical loads. The effect of SMC on restoration of the cardiorespiratory system and work capacity was studied during the preparatory period of the yearly training cycle of academic rowers. The effect of a single SMC session and a series of SMC sessions was studied. The treatments were given after the training sessions.

A total of 150 highly qualified athletes (Class I and higher) 17-20 years old were studied. One hundred and twenty of them underwent 3-4 series of 8-10 treatments each of SMC during 6 months of training (main group) with 1 month intervals. Thirty of the athletes did not undergo SMC (control group).

The treatments were conducted when the athletes were resting between two work-outs, 20-30 minutes after the first workout. Electrodes 10 x 15 cm in size were placed on the most fatigued thigh muscle. Modulation frequency was 100-

150 Hz, depth 75-100%, third and fourth type of work, current strength from 10-80 mA. The action lasted for 5 minutes for each type of work. The total duration of the treatment was 10 minutes.

The course of the restorative processes and the functional state of the body were judged from gas exchange, mechano-cardiography, myotonometry and cycle ergometry. Arterial pressure (AP) and heart rate (HR) was determined in all the athletes. Self-feeling was also taken into consideration. In the main group, maximum AP after training was 160±3.8 mm Hg. After the SMC maximum AP was 123±3.6 mm Hg (minimum AP was 63il.26 mm Hg). In the control group after training, AP was equal to 155±3.2 mm Hg, and after a 15 minute rest it was 145±3.3 mm Hg. Thus, the decrease in AP that was elevated after training was more pronounced after the SMC procedure.

Study of gas exchange made it possible to evaluate the change in the state of the aerobic and anaerobic processes of energy metabolism in the athletes according to total work, load power, maximum oxygen consumption, 'oxygen debt' and oxygen pulse. Studies were made twice a year on the Spirolit-2 under laboratory conditions after a course of SMC at the beginning of the preparatory and competitive periods of the yearly training cycle. The athletes worked on the cycle ergometer with increasing physical loads until 'refusal.'
Measurements were recorded during 5 minutes of rest, during loads, and also during the 15-20 minute restorative period (after the loads). Fifty athletes of the main and 20 of the control group were examined. It was noted that the work power, maximum oxygen consumption, 'oxygen debt' and oxygen pulse in the main group of athletes increased significantly by the beginning of the competitive period, i.e. after the SMC courses. This was evidence of increased capabilities of the aerobic and anaerobic energy processes and improvement in the functional condition of the heart. An increase in the studied factors was observed in the control group athletes, but it was less pronounced.

HR dynamics during restoration after maximal loads was also a significant factor in determining the degree of preparation of the athletes' bodies. A point scale (Skorodumova and Ozolin) was used to evaluate the changes in HR at the 5th-10th minute of the restorative period after the maximum work. At the beginning of the preparatory period, the scale reading of one athlete was 6.2, in the beginning of the competitive period, 7.5. In the control group it was 5.5 and 6.6 points, respectively, which indicated better restoration of HR in the main group of athletes.

Plastic and contractile muscle tone of the thighs and shins were studied in 55 athletes of the main and 25 of the control groups before, directly after SMC and after 30 minutes. It was found that contractile muscle tone improved under the influence of SMC, while plastic muscle tone decreased. This appeared as increased amplitude of muscle tone (difference between the contractile and plastic tone). It was 22.1±3.1 myotones in the main group after the load and 42.8±2.1 myotones after the SMC. In the control group it was 29.8±3.1 after the load and 39.2±2.9 myotones after a 15-minute rest. This shows the improved functional condition of the muscles.

Physical work capacity of 115 athletes in the main and 30 in the control group was studied after the SMC course. Physical work capacity (PWC170) in the main group of Class I athletes before and after the SMC course was 1178±34,0 and 1450±21.3 kg-m/min, respectively. Work capacity increased from 1200±25.6 to 1320iJ5.7 kg-m/min in the control group after 8-10 days of training.

Thus, our studies substantiate increased physical work capacity, improved energy processes and the functional condition of the heart, as well as accelerated restoration after physical loads in rowers receiving SMC.

Chapter 10:

DRUGS IN THE SOVIET SPORT SYSTEM

Several years ago an American athlete who was an outstanding mile runner came to me for some instruction and guidance. At that point, his best time was 3:54, and I felt he was on the brink of challenging Steve Scott and the other great U.S. milers.

As well as having films taken of his race technique, I studied his conditioning and training programs, particularly in the areas of strength and speed-strength preparation. After looking at the films, I met with his coaches and we talked for two to three hours.

I pointed out several serious flaws in the runner's technique which, if corrected, might cut his times by perhaps three seconds. I also explained the importance of adding some Soviet strengthening exercises to his workout schedule, especially for the legs and lower back, which had recently begun to bother him. Several times during that meeting, I emphasized the benefits of adjusting his program to improve his speed and speed endurance.

I felt extremely pleased as the session ended, knowing that if the young runner followed through on my recommendations, he could soon become a formidable challenger. I believe he could have been a wonderful success story.

But before leaving, one of his coaches pulled me aside and whispered, "Dr. Yessis, you and I both know that the Soviets are using superior drugs, and this is the real key to their success. I don't think their training is any different than ours, and even though you gave us some suggestions, they won't overcome the advantage that the Soviets have because of their drug use. What are the latest drugs that the Soviets are using?"

While he waited for my answer, I could only look at him in disbelief. I was not only disappointed at how misinformed he was, but I immediately realized that my recommendations would not be taken seriously.

I was right. The runner's coaches never implemented any of my suggestions. Nothing was done to improve his physical condition or running technique. "Psyched out" by phantom "perfect" drugs, the coaches were content to let their young athlete plateau at a level that I believe is considerably below his potential. At last report, he was still being clocked at about the same time in competition. What a waste!

For too many years American coaches have cited drug use as the reason for the Soviet Union's repeated victories in international meets. But they're wrong. As Chapter Two pointed out, sophisticated sports research and superior training techniques—not drugs—are the reasons for the Soviet success.

Yes, there was indeed a time when athletes in the U.S.S.R. experimented widely with drugs. The Soviets have always looked for new and different methods that might give their athletes a competitive edge, and drugs were once seen as an area worthy of exploration.

But today, the issue is much more muddled. Soviet coaches and athletes have told me stories of some athletes who continue to use these substances, but my overall impression is that the Soviets now generally perceive drugs to be counterproductive. The athletes who do take steroids tend to be the weaker, less-accomplished ones trying to make the grade. Their elite counterparts don't really feel the need for the boost that these drugs allegedly provide.

In other socialist-bloc nations, the Soviets certainly do not dictate what the athletes there do with regard to drugs. But the fear of getting caught in the growing number of drug testing programs is minimizing—or at least changing— drug use by athletes in the entire Eastern bloc.

I also learned that even those athletes who continue to consume these drugs—in the U.S.S.R. and their allied nations —take them in a unique way. They are swallowed in very small doses so that they tend to work *with* the body rather than in quantities large enough to suppress some of its most critical functions, including the production of essential hormones. These athletes take the drugs only in the early preparatory stage of their training schedule—many weeks and months before competition. By the time they move into the specialized training period, they have ceased using the drugs and are utilizing restorative techniques—including several specialized pharmacological agents—that effectively remove the illegal drugs from the athletes' systems. As a result, testing procedures over the years at the Olympic Games have caught only one Soviet athlete with drugs in his bloodstream. The fact is that in the West, our record is not nearly as good.

It is also important to emphasize that drug use among athletes appears to occur without the official sanction of coaches in the U.S.S.R. The Soviets are keenly aware of the detrimental side effects of using steroids. In contrast, I have talked to a great many American athletes who are convinced that steroids will only make them bigger, stronger, and able to train harder. Many athletes in the U.S. are either unaware of these potential problems, or have chosen to ignore them.

Thus, many thousands of athletes are jumping onto the steroid bandwagon with blinders on. As a recent statement by the Medical Commission of the International Olympic Committee observed, "The merciless rigor of modern competitive sports, especially at the international level, the glory of victory and the growing social and economic reward of sporting success . . . increasingly force athletes to improve their performance by any means possible."

As with all drugs, each individual responds differently to steroids. So while it's true that they are extremely effective for a few athletes, they are only moderately helpful for the majority. But as a result of the pressure to win at all levels of sports —from junior high school up to the professional ranks—athletes are taking enormous risks with their bodies, consuming steroids with regularity, without any careful medical monitoring along the way.

Derived from testosterone (the male hormone), the steroids that athletes take have a number of minor side effects, from oily skin to acne to increases in body hair. However, there are other, much more serious problems associated with abuse of these drugs. Though young, healthy athletes often deceive themselves into thinking they are invincible, some have experienced heart attacks, stroke, kidney damage, and liver disorders caused by consuming them. Athletes have actually died using steroids. A Bulgarian coach recently reported the death of an athlete who was regularly using 230 mg of steroids a day. In short, these drugs can kill.

Soviet research also shows that heavy use of steroids actually slows the muscles down and weakens the joints, thus leading to a poor performance and an increased risk of injury. This, apparently, is what happens with them: though steroids can lead to rapid and significant increases in muscle mass and strength, enhanced development of the support structures proceeds more slowly. Thus, the tendons and ligaments often can't withstand the new forces that the muscles exert, and injuries occur. Over time, then, steroids lead to declines in speed, endurance, and explosiveness.

Moreover, even when athletes do take drugs, they still must train. And as the Soviets have discovered, they often have to train *harder* because of the drugs they are consuming. As one of the U.S.S.R.'s top weight-lifting coaches told me, "If an athlete is stupid enough to use steroids, then *how* he trains becomes all the more important."

Soviet coaches today are insisting that their athletes avoid drugs completely, while in too many cases, American coaches are content to look the other way. As a result, Eastern-bloc weightlifters in the heavyweight division are slimmer and trimmer—not bigger and brawnier—than ever before.

Pisarenko, the Soviet's premier superheavyweight lifter in the 1980s, weighs a relatively trim 270 pounds, and has a 51-inch chest and a 36-inch waist. He believes that the key to his success has not been to be bigger, but rather to be stronger and faster. Slimmer, trimmer, faster—these are the qualities that Soviet weightlifters are seeking today.

What do the Eastern-bloc athletes use in lieu of drugs? The previous chapters of this book should help answer that question. The Soviets rely on techniques ranging from restorative approaches to nutritional programs. And obviously these seem to be working rather well.

One other drug should be mentioned. In the U.S., some American athletes are showing an interest in the so-called human growth hormone (HGH). This natural substance can make muscles larger and thicker, and in adolescents, who are still growing, it can increase their height as well.

Until recently, HGH was scarce, since it had to be extracted from the pituitary gland of cadavers. But thanks to genetic engineering, it can now be mass-produced in the laboratory.

HGH will soon be available as a prescription drug for children with serious growth problems. But I also know that parents of young athletes have already inquired of their doctors about obtaining the drug for their adolescent (and pre-adolescent) children, hoping that a little extra muscle mass will help Junior make the football team, or an extra inch or two of height will earn him a place on the basketball squad. There is already a black market for HGH in the athletic community.

Animal studies, however, have clearly shown that though large doses of HGH administered over long periods of time will result in significant growth, it exacts a price. Laboratory rats on HGH have towered over their peers, but they have been lumbering, grotesque, nonathletic, and unhealthy giants — with *a* shortened lifespan.

Consequently, research in the Soviet Union is now aimed in other directions. For instance, some scientists in the U.S.S.R. are learning to use natural stimulants already in the air which provoke certain desirable biological actions. Research has shown that the presence of these natural products is usually markedly decreased in indoor arenas and gymnasiums. Thus, efforts are being made to isolate and utilize these substances in interior settings.

Soviet researchers are particularly interested in the stimulants released from Siberian spruce, fir, and evergreen trees called alpha-pinene, beta-pinene, camphene, bornylace-tate, carene, caryophyllene, and terpinene. Early studies show they are capable of beneficially stimulating activity in the cardiovascular and other systems, especially during intensive workouts. The oxidative processes of the heart are intensified, the heart rate declines, blood pressure normalizes, and thermal discomfort is minimized.

The Soviets hope to improve the indoor air environments of gymnasiums and arenas with these substances. It certainly seems to make more sense to rely on these natural stimulants than the synthetic, illegal drugs used by so many athletes. I hope we in the West will follow suit and move *beyond* drugs and into other areas of sports training; as this book emphasizes, it is possible to train effectively without resorting to illegal substances. You can be drug-free and still be a winner.

TABLE 13 Distribution of Time of Training Loads and Special Means of Restoration in the Weekly Cycle of Preparation (Min)

Training Load and Means of Restoration	Days of the Week							Weekly Total
	1	2	3	4	5	6	7	
Training load:								
morning	45	45	45	45	45	45	45	315
daytime	150	90	120	—	150	90	—	600
evening	90	—	90	—	90	90	—	360
General physical preparation	30	60	30	90	30	60	60	360
Total for the day	315	195	285	135	315	285	105	1635
Means of restoration:								
hand massage		30				30		60
vibrational massage	15		30		20			65
"electrical" vibro-bath		20						20
contrast baths		5				5		10
water showers	10	5	10	10	10	5	10	60
Sharko shower		5				5		10
flowing stream shower		5				5		10
ultraviolet irradiation		5		5		5		15
heat bath (sauna)*		15				15		30
pine needle baths	10			10				20
psychorehabilitation**	30				30			60
Total for the day (min.):	65	90	40	25	60	70	10	360

*Time actually in heat room.
**Includes simultaneous use of low-frequency vibromassage, psychoregulatory training, musical and light influences.

Chapter 10 Addendum

The information presented in the original text can now be somewhat clarified. In the intervening years I have talked to several high level Russian coaches who have corroborated and filled in more details on what I had written. They did not dispute the use of steroids by athletes but they were emphatic in stating that the amount of steroid use was practically nothing in comparison to what athletes are presently taking in the U.S. and other countries. When they used steroids it was only for a two week period as a boost in the preparatory period and in small dosages. There were, however, abuses by some athletes.

The Russians, through their research and practical use of steroids, know (as athletes have also discovered) that they are effective in improving performance. For example, if you compare two athletes--one who trains without drugs and another who trains in exactly the same manner with the same exercises and same exercise routine but uses steroids you will see a distinct difference. The athlete who trained without the use of drugs will show gains in all of the exercises. However, the athlete using steroids will show greater gains in the exercises and in his performance. This is well established. Athletes know it can improve performance.

According to the coaches, the problem with using steroids, is that although you can get by with a relatively small amount in the first year, in the next and following years the amount needed for the same results keeps increasing. Very soon the dosages are very big and the negative effects happen very quickly.

These negative effects, some of which are not well known in the U.S. include: Technique of skill execution changes which in turn interferes with the ability of the athlete to execute his skills well, thus diminishing his performance. There is a greater incidence of injury, that holds back the athletes progress. As a result, even though an athlete not using drugs shows smaller gains, he will be able to train on a more consistent basis making gains, which over several years, will be greater than the athlete using steroids.

In regard to injury, it is well known that although the use of steroids leads to increases in muscle strength and mass, the tendons lag behind. This results in an imbalance between muscle and tendon strength. When the muscle becomes much stronger and contracts at maximum intensity, an injury is almost unavoidable to the tendon or muscle—tendon junction. This is why it is not uncommon to see many injuries in which the muscle tendon rips off the bone. This is seen in many bodybuilders and in an increasing number of athletes.

The negative side effects of steroid use especially in regard to body health are well known, but the kinds of injuries and what bodily changes take place vary greatly depending upon the athlete. For example, 'roid rage' is very common with some athletes while others only become more aggressive in their workouts. Some begin to experience cardiovascular problems, more specifically heart problems, or skin, kidney and other organ disruptions. A number of male athletes lose their ability to reproduce while with others it seems to have little effect. In any case, the athlete is playing "Russian roulette" with his life, well being and athletic career. It is a shame that many athletes who have used steroids do not come clean and tell other athletes about the negative effects that they have experienced.

With the use of steroids, especially in high doses, and especially with "stacking", i.e. using several or more different concoctions at the same time athletes, may experience fame and glory. But it will be short lived. For example, Marion Jones had great success in the Olympics in which she won five medals. However, since that time she was not able to reproduce any of her outstanding achievements. Know we know she was a steroid user and even with all she was taking, she could not repeat or surpasses her best one time results. The exact reasons for this are unknown. It appears to be definitely related to the changes that took place with the steroids. If she had trained naturally with the great athletic talent which I believe she had, she could have reproduced the same or even better results in the ensuing years—especially if she had trained wisely with scientific methods.

Even in baseball there are examples of home run hitters such as Roger Maris having success with steroids. But, after breaking the home run record, he was no longer capable of reproducing this feat. Because of his injuries and other problems, he was soon no longer able to play. Others who have been accused of using drugs, or in cases where it is fairly well established that they used drugs but not yet proven, as for example, Barry Bonds, we can see many physical problems and the inability to reproduce even close to the same number of home runs as in the record year.

In these cases, it is not just the steroids that hold back further progress but the player's inability to execute game skills as effectively as he or she could have or once was capable of doing But, since baseball is so far behind in the use of science no one has seriously looked at the technique of these performers and what changes have taken place over the years. If they did they would see some dramatic differences.

It also appears that EPO is being used with increasing frequency in the endurance events, especially in cycling. In the past few years several cyclists have been caught using EPO during the Tour de France and other events. Several were even busted this year during the Tour de France even though they knew they would be tested. Still other athletes have been caught in different endurance sporting events such as the triathlon.

To help stop drug use by athletes, many teams and organizations are now requiring that the athletes be tested on a sometimes regular, or irregular basis. This is a good deterrent but unless the testing is done without the athletes knowing that they will be tested and when they will be tested, athletes can easily prepare for it. Thus, it may not be as strong a deterrent as it could be.

Compounding the problem and I believe helping to perpetuate drug use by athletes, is the media. The reason for this is simple. The media does not look at player development. By this I mean what is behind player performance and only sensationalize the fact that some players are or were users or were reported to have used steroids or other drugs. To them, this is big news and they can't wait to make the most of it.

They do not write about player skills or how effectively they are executed during game play. They have little if any comprehension of the relationship between player skills and the ability to perform well on the field. Because of this it is understandable that they can only write about the obvious and do not have the ability to do any true investigative reporting. But this is still no excuse for not trying to take a look at the total picture.

It is great that they report on who was or is using drugs, how they were caught, how long they were using, etc. But this side of drug use should be balanced by articles showing the negative effects of steroids and how athletes, if they trained scientifically and used some of the latest and best methods, could get the same if not better results without the use of steroids. But the media does not consider itself as a source of such information and appears to refuse to publish any articles that may sound "educational".

By sensationalizing drug use the media in essence are saying that "successful", or perhaps accomplished is a better term, athletes use steroids. This implies that if you want to be great you must use steroids. Even in the past when it was proven that the East Germans were into drugs, there were many stories dealing with this topic. But, there were no articles dealing with any aspects of the East German (or Russian on which the East German system was based) training system. All the articles dealt with the athletes using drugs and this was the reason for their success. This was and is far from the truth.

For some reason the sports media believes that coaches already do an effective job of not only developing players but fully exploiting their potential. But as brought out, they do not. Youth leagues, high schools, and collegiate league teams are all set up for athletes to play against one another. They are set up to determine winners and losers, not to see who can develop into the best athlete. This is why professional, collegiate and to a good extent high school, teams rely so heavily on recruiting to get the best players to fill the best teams.

If you look closely at collegiate and professional teams, you will see that a high percentage of the athletes are foreign. Having some is understandable and good for the sport, but up to 50% or more foreign players is not. This is indicative of the inability to develop athletic talent. Professional and top collegiate teams travel the world over to find what they consider to be the best talent. This shows that they cannot improve an athlete's performance except in the area of strategy and tactics. They are not able to get the athletes to execute better skills or improve their technical and physical abilities to better carry out the strategies desired by the coaches. As a result, athletes are still not able to execute their skills in a reliable and consistent fashion.

This is not surprising. Coaches keep analyzing their strategy and even go to great lengths to spy on teams to find out what other teams are doing so that they can more effectively strategize against them. But they do not use proven scientific and practical methods to improve the physical and technical aspects of player performance. Greatest value is given to recruiting, collegiate and high school drafts and buying at the professional level. There are even organizations whose main function is to trace the development of a particular athlete in relation to his wins and losses and how well he is expected to do. Teams rely heavily on these reports for their recruiting efforts.

Collegiate teams spend millions of dollars on recruiting every year but not a penny on player development as previously defined. Professional teams spend mega millions on buying athletes and developing training facilities in foreign countries, but do not spend money on player development or even similar facilities in the U.S. Minor league teams for feeding players into the major leagues are set up not to develop physical and technical abilities, but to allow for more playing time, strategy work and rehabilitation, hoping that a few gems will be discovered.

Based on what the Russians experienced, if drug use is to be minimized greatly in the U.S. and hopefully, eventually eliminated, it will take more than just athletic organizations condemning the use of steroids or establishing programs for the prevention of drug use. It will take the influence of the media to get the word out to the entire population. In addition, coaches who are parents have to be educated on the effects of steroids and other drugs especially as they relate to sports performance. The medical aspects of steroid and other drug use have been well documented and written up many times. However, studies have shown that knowing the negative health effects of steroids is not an effective deterrent. Athletes still use them because they would rather achieve fame and glory in spite of what it might do to their body, health and future careers.

When the media popularizes effective and scientifically proven training methods that can truly develop athletic talent and improve athletic performance, then we may see athletes not using drugs. Until then, the media, by sensationalizing drugs, merely perpetuate the myth that athletes need drugs in order to succeed.

Sports magazines such as *Sports Illustrated*, that have an extensive following in the U.S., should also help prevent drug use. Sadly however, they appear to be more interested in writing about athlete personalities and creating celebrities rather than being concerned about whether they use drugs or how they train.

For example, when I trained Todd Marinovich, football quarterback, who broke all the high school records for passing, etc., *Sports Illustrated* did a major feature article on him. Since I was the main specialist working with Todd and who directed his training, I talked to the writer at length for a few hours about the unique methods of training that I used with Todd. Many of these methods were based on Russian techniques that were never before used in the U.S. After our discussion he seemed quite impressed and stated he would definitely write about them. However, when the article came out, not one word was said about the training that Todd did. Instead we read about his not eating any Twinkies and other junk foods and how his parents regulated his food intake, lifestyle and social life.

When I called and asked the reporter why he didn't say anything about his training, his reply was short and direct, "Coaches already know how to train an athlete". With attitudes such as this, we will never see any real changes that could benefit athletes and the country as a whole. Instead we will see more articles dealing with the celebrity status of athletes and more about their sex and social lives rather than their playing performance.

It appears that sports reporters will continue to act as parrots for the players and teams by merely repeating the statements that they make in locker rooms and in press conferences before and after games. There is no investigative reporting in the area of sports. The only exception may be the reporting by the San Francisco Chronicle reporters on drug use in athletics. Until then, it appears that the media will keep their blinders on and only sensationalize drugs.

Chapter 11:

WHAT'S ON THE HORIZON?

By now, this book should have made clear why it is that athletes from the U.S.S.R. so consistently outperform their peers from other countries in international meets. A superior training system—supported by the most sophisticated sports research program in the world— continues to bring home the gold to the Soviet Union year after year.

But what about the future? Are the Soviets destined to maintain their superiority, thanks to even newer techniques already being developed and scrutinized by some of the best scientific minds behind the Iron Curtain?

In each of my trips to the U.S.S.R., I have come away convinced that the Soviets are not about to yield their supremacy in the world of sports. Chances are good that the Eastern-bloc countries will remain as innovative in the future as they have been in the past.

Take the field of biomechanics, for example. Essentially, this is the study of movement during sports performance. With careful scrutiny, scientists can determine the best technique for a sprinter, the most effective way for a high jumper to kick during his takeoff, or the techniques that will help a hammer thrower avoid injuries.

One of the keys to this kind of investigation is the measurement of the movements of athletes without interfering with them. The fact is that no one does this better than the Soviets. They currently have the most advanced stereo-photographic, optico-electronic, laser, and telemetric registration techniques anywhere in the world.

They are currently integrating all these elements into a single unit that, when fully operational, will completely eclipse the capabilities of any other system on the horizon. Imagine a gymnasium equipped with a series of high-speed videotape cameras placed around the room, and electronic registration devices inserted in the walls. The floors will contain sensing devices that take an array of measurements each time the foot touches the ground. These will determine exactly how long the foot is in contact with the ground, how long the runner is airborne, and the force exerted horizontally and vertically. At the same time, lasers will instantly calculate the speed and acceleration of each part of the athlete's body (see Figure 43),

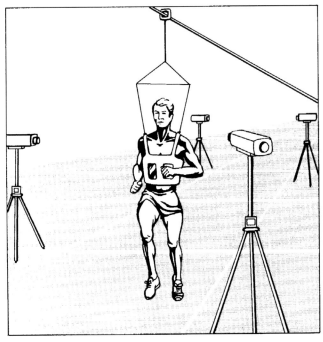

Figure 43.

All these data will be automatically channeled into a computer, which will analyze them in seconds, identify any imperfections, and suggest precisely how to correct them. It's a coach's—and an athlete's—dream.

The Soviets are designing a number of other intriguing training aids, too. Robots, for example, are being developed for use as "training partners" for fencers, judoists, and wrestlers, allowing these athletes to practice certain movements and reactions against a "perfect" opponent.

Some practitioners of judo are already using a robot as their part-time sparring partner. Covered by leather, its interior is a complex mesh of electronic apparatus that includes a computer, four programs, and the capacity to be controlled by radio. Figure 44, reprinted from a Soviet sports journal, shows both the exterior and the interior of one of these robots.

Other futuristic techniques are also already being used in the U.S.S.R. Fingerprints, for instance, may not seem to have many applications in athletics, but in fact they do behind the Iron Curtain. Research has found that the fingerprints of the fourth and fifth fingers of the left hand can be used to determine present flexibility and the potential for flexibility in the future. Weightlifters and gymnasts are finding this technique especially useful in devising a workout program for improving flexibility.

The Soviets are also experimenting with electronic equipment capable of measuring "electro-skin resistance." It is being used with athletes in a growing number of sports to evaluate precompetitive emotional excitation. Researchers have learned that levels of excitation can influence performance to a great extent. The most outstanding athletes have a high and stable level of emotional excitation before competition, compared to a wide range of fluctuation or variability in less-successful athletes. Once an individual has been evaluated, techniques have been used to regulate these precompetition emotional states, ranging from self-suggestion to specialized exercises.

To develop explosiveness, the Soviets are also experimenting with attaching athletes to devices capable of transmitting subtle electrical stimulation. A shot-putter, for instance, is hooked up to this apparatus during some of his training sessions, and as he goes through the movements of his event, he is subjected to electrical current just before he releases the shot. Studies show that, as a result, the shot is propelled with more explosive power.

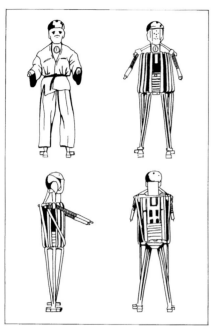

Figure 44.

The theory behind this approach is based on the idea that as the athlete experiences higher and higher speed, his central nervous system is learning precisely how that speed is achieved. Ultimately, his arm will move more quickly on its own—and he'll achieve more explosiveness—after the electrical stimulation is removed.

The Soviet coaches also spend a great deal of time helping their athletes get in touch with their own bodies and assess their capabilities on a particular day. I recall, during one of my visits, a top weightlifting coach explained that when his lifters worked out, they could sense after just a few warmup lifts how much they'd be able to lift that day with a given exercise. This is called "instinctive training," and it can take an athlete many years to perfect it.

The technique requires that the athlete become sensitive to the nerve endings and other receptors that send messages to the brain about what is occurring within the muscles, tendons, and joints. Over a period of time, the individual develops the concentration that allows him or her to listen to his or her body, and become aware of its signals and messages. You, too, can eventually learn to recognize what your body is telling you, and then adjust the intensity of your workout accordingly.

If you are sensitive to your body, you should notice any deviations from the way you normally perform bench presses, for example. An arch in the back or a slight variation in the angle of your arms should be warning signs to stop or to make necessary adjustments. An unfamiliar ache or pain in the muscles or joints is a signal that an injury may have occurred, and steps should be taken to prevent further damage.

At the suggestion of Soviet coaches, I now have many of the American athletes I work with keep a detailed diary of their workouts. They not only keep track of the exercises performed, the number of repetitions and the weight used, but they also make notes about what they felt and experienced during the exercise routines. Over a period of six months to a year, they become proficient at interpreting and applying the messages they receive during their workouts.

While Soviet athletes develop and refine techniques like these, they are supported by a system that considers sports as a national treasure. As we have noted, and as Table 14 documents, sports have become a crucial aspect of Soviet life, and its growth continues to be phenomenal.

TABLE 14 Development of Sports in the Soviet Union, 1964 to 1980

	1964	1980
Regular participants in physical culture and sports	43 million	82 million
Preparation of athletes:		
Master of sport	8,900	12,200
Candidates for Class I athlete	95,500	469,300
Athletes in the mass ranks	7 million	25 million
Number of sports buildings:		
Sports gyms	26,500	74,200
Swimming pools	700	1,700
Sports courts and fields	396,800	541,100
Trained public inspectors and coaches	2 million	10 million
Trained sports judges and referees	2 million	7 million
Participants in the sports sections in schools	38 million	46 million

I also continue to be amazed at how differently athletes are treated in the East and the West. I sometimes explain this difference by using a metaphor that equates an elite athlete with a Rolls-Royce. In the U.S., we treat our best athletes like Rolls-Royces, glorying in their quality, but we leave these Rolls-Royces parked in the driveway, to be spattered by rain and snow, and driven mile after mile without receiving even the most basic maintenance such as lubrication and oil changes. Yes, we fill them up with gas, but when one breaks down we just discard it and get another.

By contrast, in the U.S.S.R., coaches have never felt that they have a base of outstanding athletes so large that they could care for them poorly. Thus, much as a prized Rolls-Royce should be treated, athletes there are nurtured with tender loving care. They receive the best coaching that is available in their area. These youngsters are encouraged in every way possible to reach their full potential. The nation's top athletes —e.g., the Mary Lou Rettons of the U.S.S.R.—frequently tour Soviet schools and athletic clubs, inspiring younger, newer competitors to reach even greater heights.

There's another powerful motive for this strong emphasis on sports, of course. When Soviet athletes perform well in international meets, it is perceived as a victory for socialism. Thus, there is a strong political impetus to succeed in the arena of sports, for more is at stake than personal objectives. One observer of the U.S.S.R. has written, "The Soviets have made serious business out of sports competition. It has become a war without employing the tools of war."

No one knows just how far the Soviet Union's sophisticated sports system will take its athletes. As you've learned in this book, they already are innovators in fields such as explosiveness training, speed-strength exercises, aerobic fitness, nutrition, and restoration. Most observers have stopped trying to project just how high they can raise the ceilings on sports records, recognizing that these marks have been raised time and time again, and that this will probably continue to occur. Rather than there being a slowdown in record-breaking performances as man approaches his hypothetical limits, the opposite seems to be true: the higher the world marks go, the quicker they seem to be broken.

In the 1980 Olympic Games in Moscow, for instance, there were eighteen world records broken in weightlifting alone. (By comparison, no new records were set in the Olympics in Los Angeles four years later, where no Eastern-bloc lifters competed.) After those amazing performances in Moscow, it seemed logical that a lull would occur in record-breaking performances. But that didn't happen. In the 1983 world and European weightlifting championships, twenty-three new world records were set. The sky really does seem to be the limit.

Fortunately, the Soviets are more than willing to share their innovative sports training techniques. As one coach said, "We want to compete against the world's best. And your athletes in America can be even better than they already are."

I agree. In the U.S., our athletes—as talented and proficient as they currently are—still have enormous room for improvement. It will take some restructuring of the way we approach sports. But the talented young athletes we have here in the U.S. deserve all the help that research, innovative techniques, and sports laboratories of our own could give them.

If we began to take sports science and apply it at all levels as seriously as the Soviets do, and take advantage of all the intricate information that it can uncover, I believe we could eventually go head to head with the Soviets in international competition and come out the winner. I'm looking forward to that day.

Chapter 11 Addendum

In regard to what's on the horizon and what's going on in Russia at present, a few changes are becoming very visible. It appears that the government is now taking a greater interest in sports as putting more money back into the programs especially into facilities. The increase in money has been quite substantial. According to some sources they have gone from a few hundred thousand dollars in some areas and over $1 billion in others. Some of this new money has come from rich oilmen especially in the construction of new facilities.

This is similar to what has taken place in the United States as for example, ARCO donating $60 million to establish an Olympic training Center in San Diego. However, the U.S. Olympic Committee and private donors have not come up with additional monies to make this center fully functional. This may also happen in Russian if the new monies are only put into facilities.

If even more money is put into expanding the Sports Research Institute, coaching institutes and sports schools, it will help greatly in bringing back the very successful sports programs as seen in the past. Thus, there may be substantial a resurrection of the old system or modifications of it. However, it should be noted that even though the original system is gone, there are still ample remnants of it still in place. Research is still being done, training methods are being analyzed, training systems are being looked at more closely and innovations are on the horizon.

Most changes that I see happening could take place in the United States (and in other countries) to develop the athletic programs. We already have better technology, more athletes, more equipment, better facilities and more private support for sport than any other country in the world. In spite of this, we are not developing the best athletes. We have some of the best athletes, but most of these athletes come from the mass numbers of participants, not because of the best training methods.

If the best training were coupled with the largest number of athletes, we would have the most powerful sports system in the world. There will always be exceptions in certain sports but by and large, a greater dominance would given to the United States. However, I do not see this happening in the very near future in spite of all the advantages that we presently possess. We are still not looking closely at how to improve specific physical and technical abilities of athletes—the key to executing skills well which are the cornerstone of any great athlete.

For example, in relation to technology, companies duplicated some of the equipment depicted in the original text. One example is the apparatus on which the athlete is lifted up so that the body becomes lighter which then allows him to run faster. However, when I saw this apparatus and how it was used, it was obvious that the company knew little about the training of a sprinter and was merely out to sell the machine. It did not appear that they were interested in how the runner should be trained using the machine together with other trainings. It was a classic example of great technology but not knowing what to do with it.

There are even some television programs today that feature sports science but they are more show than substance. The material that they present is excellent. They report and show what some athletes are capable of doing but they show nothing about how such talent can be developed. They usually select a top player in the sport and just test or measure the athlete to show his capabilities. They measure how much force he exerts, how high he can jump, how fast he can run, etc. But, nothing is shown in regard to how the physical quality is developed or even if other people can develop this ability and how.

There are even programs in which baseball myths are exposed. They have done some excellent work in this area but how concepts can be changed and what should be done in training in relation to the myth that was broken, is not addressed. For example, there was discussion about what makes a ball curve or deviate from a straight line path. They used a wind tunnel with some dust particles that were illuminated and then recorded the air currents that developed around the ball as it traveled through the air. It was great for understanding what happens to the ball in flight. But they did not show the path of a particular pitch.

They only used one pitcher and his description of what constitutes a curveball. But yet, in the baseball world, this definition is not universally accepted. They assumed that everyone understands what a curveball, breaking ball and slider is. It's just another example of the myths that are perpetuated in baseball and other sports. We're not using technology to clarify and explain exactly what each pitch is, the pathway that it takes, and more importantly, how it is thrown. Very few if any have actually looked at the mechanics of throwing different pitches. This is where technology can play a very important role.

To do this, there must be greater use of biomechanics which in this content means analysis of sports technique. The bio prefix refers to biological aspects while mechanics refers to the physical (physics) or technical aspects of the movement. In the US we usually use the term kinesiology to describe the biological aspects or more specifically, the muscle and joint involvement. In either case, when technique is analyzed we should look at it from all sides to determine exactly which muscles are involved, how they're involved, how the levers are moved, what happens in the joint, how the action can be made more effective, what constitutes effective skill execution, how the skill can be improved, and so on. These are the questions that only biomechanics can answer.

Sadly however, we do not have coaches with such biomechanical expertise nor do we have professors at the university with this expertise. A few professors and researchers on the university level do some outstanding quantitative work in the area of biomechanics. They can describe in detail the mechanics of the execution. However, they cannot answer how effective the movement is, how it could be improved, what could make it better and so on. This is what should be added to the work that is being done.

In addition, many of the biomechanical studies are done with novice athletes and the results then applied to all level athletes. However, this is not accurate. We need a greater library of different athletes and their technique execution recorded in order to come up with effective technique for the multitude of athletes.

Just as each athlete is different physically, their technique will also be different. Also important in this regard is to use biomechanics to correct or enhance technique. This is a very critical and important area. Many coaches are capable of bringing out some technique flaws but are not capable of understanding what causes the flaw or how it can be corrected, especially through specialized strength exercises.

This would be a great area of innovation in the US but it will take a concentrated effort on the part of both university professors and coaches to develop specialists in this area. They must be willing to learn more to help improve the athletes.

In the last few years before the breakup of the USSR, the Russians were developing methods to monitor all systems of the athlete in order to better direct the training process. The monitoring was done on various levels with fairly sophisticated equipment that measured heart performance, oxygen utilization, inter and intra cellular water levels as well as many indicators in the blood of what is transpiring in the various organs and systems of the body. With this feedback, it was possible to know exactly what changes are taking place in the body from the workout and also to figure out what kind of workout should be done on the following day (based on body system function).

Some of these monitoring systems are now available in the U.S. and other countries. To date, they have not received wide distribution and use. The technology exists, it is only a matter of implementing and using it. But again, it takes coaches who understand the scientific bases of training and know how to incorporate the results into the training sessions.

Also new on the horizon is the use of vibrational machines and devices. These were used for many years in Russia, mainly as a means of increasing flexibility and partially for use in healing and recovery. Only in recent years has the use of vibrational machines been popularized in the US and can now be found in many fitness clubs as well as athletic facilities. But, as with many other devices that become popular, the claims for their benefits are often exaggerated and exactly how they should be used is not precise nor substantiated by the research. However, vibrational devices show great potential, but more research is needed before they can be effectively used by different populations.

There is still much to be learned about the use of electrical stimulation. This modality originated in the former Soviet Union and with American technology, many of these devices have been improved upon greatly. They have proven their value not only in development of muscle strength, but also in recovery and treatment of injury. However, there is still much to be desired in this area and more work needs to be done.

As brought out in the original text, we have not been able to find a company interested in developing an apparatus that can stimulate the muscle at the exact moment that it comes into play in execution of a sports skill. Thus, there has not been any progress in this area.

When we think in terms of what is on the horizon, we should also look closely at identification of athletes and how they respond to various training exercises and regimes. According to the Russian coaches, this appears to be a critical element in determining how effective a training program is. For example, according to Bondarchuk, the sign of a great coach is one who is capable of changing his methods according to the needs of the athlete. In other words, the coach does not merely persist in a training program that was successful in developing a world class athlete. He learns to make adjustments for different levels and types of athletes in order to bring out the best in them. This is an area that I believe needs further exploration especially in most of the popular sports.

My comments in regard to the treatment of an athlete as being analogous to taking care of a Rolls Royce still hold true today. Elite athletes can be put on the level of a Rolls Royce. But the loving care that is usually given to these high priced and beautiful cars, is not commensurate with the care given to elite athletes. Instead of looking at the athlete's training and how his or her performance can be enhanced and maintained we appear to be more concerned with making the athlete a celebrity. This is what the press pushes for: they cannot merely report the news without creating a hero or making someone into a celebrity.

Thus, the celebrity athlete becomes the focal point of many articles. For example, in any major golf tournament even if Tiger Woods is not playing, the headline may state that Tiger is not playing and therefore the tournament is now diminished in stature. If an unknown golfer wins the tournament, the stories relate to Tiger losing rather than a story about who won and more information about him. There is less press given to the winner than there is to the loser if he or she is a celebrity.

This probably explains why in many different sports we read about the same people on a constant basis. It may also explain why the payments for winning are often so distorted. Winners can make a million dollars while 3rd or 4th place may only make 50 or $100,000. It appears that if you do not take first place, you do not place in the money.

It may be time to pressure the media to give more attention to up and coming athletes and to talk more about player development. In this way they will not be obsessed with only the top celebrity. It will help greatly in terms of expanding and improving the athletic base that is needed for continued success in all sports. But if we are more interested in being spectators and only ogling at the elite or celebrity athlete, then of course, we should forget about player development. We only have to continue traveling around the world to bring in the best athletes. In my opinion this will be a throwback to the days of the gladiator. Bring on the athletes and we will have the spectators yelling, screaming and carrying on. But yet, the spectators will have no concept of what it takes to attain a high level of performance and will only be interested in winning or losing. Perhaps we have already arrived at this state in some sports.

We can say it is a shame to see the advances in the sports sciences slow down and stop in regard to the development of athletes in present day Russia and in some of the republics that broke off from the former Soviet Union. But yet, to be successful in sports, especially in countries with a small athletic base (or small market teams), there is still work to be done in this area. The Russian Sports Institutes are still conducting and reporting on research that is bringing out new concepts. If it continues, we may see additional innovations coming out of Russia.

In conclusion, I believe it may be important to re-read the last two paragraphs of the original text. They hold as true today as they did then. I hope that they will trigger greater interest and that more people will become involved and concerned about what is presently taking place in the United States. Only in this way can we truly do justice to our youth and future sports programs.

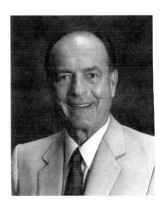

About the Author

Dr. Yessis is the foremost expert on the Russian sports training system. He has been translating Soviet/Russian books and articles for over 50 years. In addition, he has been to the Soviet Union several times and worked with their scientists and coaches as well as performing translation services and information exchanges during the former USA-USSR Track and Field meets. For over 29 years he published Russian sports training articles in the *Soviet Sports Review*, later known as the *Fitness and Sports Review International*. Dr. Yessis also wrote many articles about Russian training methods in various general and sports specific magazines.

Some of the Russian books translated include: *Transfer of Training in Sports* by Dr. Anatoly Bondarchuk, probably the most successful Olympic coach in history, and *Special Strength Training* by Dr.Yuri Verkhoshansky, the creator of plyometrics which is now a popular training method in the US. In addition, he edited *Block Periodization* by Dr.Vladimir Issurin. This book describes the latest and most important training method being used by elite and professional athletes.

Dr. Michael Yessis received his Ph.D. from the University of Southern California and his B.S. and M.S. from City University of New York. He is president of Sports Training, Inc., a diverse sports and fitness company. Dr. Yessis is also Professor Emeritus at California State University, Fullerton, where he is a multi-sports specialist in biomechanics (technique analysis) and sports conditioning and training.

In his work, Dr. Yessis has developed many unique specialized strength and speed-strength (explosive) training programs. He has served as training and technique consultant to several Olympic and professional sports teams, including the L.A. Rams and L.A. Raiders football clubs, Natadore Diving Team, and the U.S. Men's Volleyball Team. He has also successfully trained many athletes in different sports.

Dr. Yessis has written 16 books including *Kinesiology of Exercise, Explosive Running, Build A Better Athlete, and Sports: Is It All B.S.?* He has also written more than 2,000 articles on fitness and sports training that have appeared in magazines such as Muscle and Fitness, Shape, Scholastic Coach, Fitness Management, and the National Strength and Conditioning Association Journal. In addition, he has completed four videos/DVDs; Exercise Mastery, Developing a Quarterback's Arm and Strength, Specialized Strength and Explosive Exercises for Baseball and Specialized Strength and Explosive Exercises for Softball.

OTHER BOOKS BY DR. YESSIS

Build a Better Athlete

This book by Dr. Yessis is the **most comprehensive sports training book ever written** on what it takes to develop an athlete. It covers technique of the basic skills, the physical qualities needed for sports in general, for specific sports, and how they should be developed. In addition, specific recommendations on nutrition –that have never before been presented to athletes—are given in easy to understand terms. There is also a chapter on the role of vision and vision training.

The book is a culmination of over 50 years of working with and teaching athletes how to develop their full potential and be successful in their chosen sport. It is unmatched in not only it's scope, but in the detail given to each of the factors. Many of the concepts presented are **state-of-the-art and have been proven** in practice. In fact, the information is based not only on the knowledge available in the U.S. but from what has been gleaned from advanced Russian techniques.

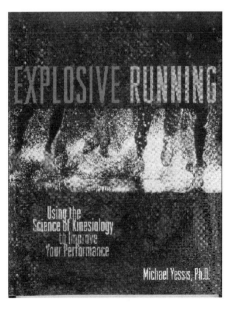

Explosive Running

This book is a book of firsts not seen in any other running book! If you have ever wanted to improve your running, there has never been a better time to start. Explosive Running is the answer to your running woes. Not only does this book explain the mechanics of running, but it breaks down running technique into easy to follow steps. No other book comes close to matching the specificity of the running technique analyses and the specialized strength and explosive exercises presented in this book. Also covered are Active stretches, barefoot running, how to fix common problems, nutrition specific to running and how to set up and conduct the workout program. Serious sprinters, long distance and running athletes in other sports should not be without it.

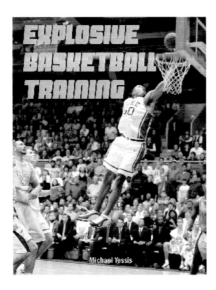

Explosive Basketball Training

The most complete book on how to become a great basketball player. This is the only book that looks at technique and special strength and explosive exercises specific to each basketball skill. In this book you will learn how to jump higher and quicker, how to shoot further and with more accuracy, how to make your cuts sharper and more powerful to become even quicker in your movements and how to run faster.

SPORTS: Is it all B.S.?

Sports: Is It All B.S.?, is an expose of the many myths and false information that have surrounded sports in the U.S. for many decades. This book is a great read for everyone interested in sports and a must read for anyone who has an athlete in the family, especially if the athlete would like to develop his or her full potential. The information appeals to not only people who are interested in sports, but to the nation as a whole. It has ramifications regarding our participation in World and Olympic Games.

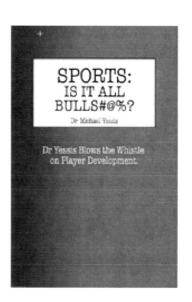

Explosive Plyometrics

Available October 2008

This will be the most up to date a book on plyometrics with information never before published in the US. Not only is plyometrics discussed, explained and illustrated it also contains information from Dr. Yuri Verkhoshansky, who is considered to be the father of plyometrics. The information includes chapters devoted to explosive arm training, explosive leg training, explosive midsection training and explosive total body training.

OTHER BOOKS AVAILABLE FROM ULTIMATE ATHLETE CONCEPTS

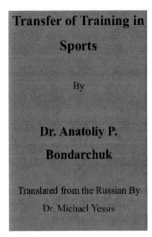

Transfer of Training in Sport

by Anatoly Bondarchuk

Translated by Dr. Michael Yessis

Transfer of Training is the first definitive book on what transfer of training is and what is involved to truly enhance performance with the use of specific exercises. Based on 10 years of study of the highest level athletes, Dr. Bondarchuk brings out which commonly used "specific" exercises truly enhance performance in throwing, jumping and running, and general principles such as conjugated effects.

Block Periodization

by Dr. Vladimir Issurin

Newly edited in English, *Block Periodization* is a revolutionary book that should be read by all coaches and athletes. *Block Periodization* is a very effective method of developing one or two physical qualities to either enhance performance or to bring up the lagging areas. It is the method for athletes who must compete most of the year.

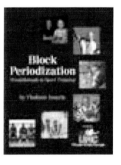

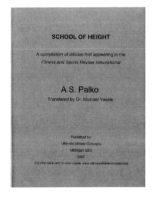

School of Height

by A.S. Palko

A compilation of articles first appearing in the *Fitness and Sports Review International*.

If you want to get taller this is the book for you. Written by A.S.Palko, renowned Russian orthopedist, this book covers the key factors involved in growing taller. In addition it tells you how various factors can be corrected and/or enhanced.